# Biochemistry of the Eye

# Biochemistry of the Eye

## David R. Whikehart, Ph.D.

*Professor*
*Vision Science Research Center*
*School of Optometry*
*The University of Alabama at Birmingham*
*Birmingham, Alabama*

**Butterworth–Heinemann**
Boston   London   Oxford   Singapore   Sydney   Toronto   Wellington

**Library of Congress Cataloging-in-Publication Data**
Whikehart, David R.
Biochemistry of the eye / David R. Whikehart.
p.  cm.
Includes index.
ISBN 0-7506-9074-7 (alk. paper)
1. Eye—Molecular aspects.    I. Title.
[DNLM: 1. Eye—chemistry.   2. Eye—physiopathology.
WW 101 W5616 1994]
QP475.W48      1994
612.8′4—dc20
DNLM/DLC
for Library of Congress                                              94-7076
                                                                         CIP


**British Library Cataloguing-in-Publication Data**

A catalogue record for this book is available from the British Library.

Butterworth-Heinemann
313 Washington Street
Newton, MA 02158-1626

10  9  8  7  6  5  4  3  2  1

Printed in the United States of America

This book is dedicated to my students: past, present, and future. They have been and will continue to be a gauge of their own success and my personal incentive for improvement.

# Contents

# Anatomical Cross Reference

# Preface

*Biochemistry of the Eye* is an effort to bring ocular biochemistry, as a subject in its own right, to the forefront. After teaching ocular biochemistry for several years, it became frustrating not to have a compact source of pertinent information on this subject. Certainly, this frustration has been shared by many students as well.

In organizing this text, the question arose about whether to format it along the lines of traditional biochemical texts, with emphasis on biochemical classes of compounds such as proteins and lipids, or whether to discuss the biochemistry of each anatomical subdivision of the eye such as the cornea and retina. The former approach was chosen since much ocular biochemistry is the same in all tissues of the eye, just as it is in all cellular biochemistry. This mode avoids redundancy. By choosing biochemical subdivisions, the opportunity presented itself to discuss general biochemistry and to include material that is peculiar to specific ocular tissues. For example, under proteins, one can include the globular proteins present everywhere in tissues as well as lens crystallins and retinal rhodopsin. Anyone who may wish to take the opposite route is at liberty to use the cross-reference in the early section of this book in order to learn that biochemistry which is particular to each anatomical subdivision of the eye.

Efforts have been made to use many concise but inclusive illustrations of biochemical classes, their interactions, and their locations in ocular tissues. The text itself is meant to guide the reader to meaningful conclusions about the subject. For that purpose the text is well integrated with the illustrations.

Where possible, many examples of biochemical pathology and disease processes have been described. The reader will find, in particular, rather extensive descriptions of age-related cataract formation and ocular diabetes. It is hoped that these will be meaningful when students advance to courses in ocular pathology. The biochemical foundations of many ocular physiological processes and pharmacological applications have also been included, to give needed professional breadth to the subject.

All these efforts reflect a sincere wish to heighten the student's awareness of the molecular structures and biochemical events that occur in the eye. For readers who are receptive, *Biochemistry of the Eye* should enhance their professional training.

David R. Whikehart

# Acknowledgments

I am happy to acknowledge the dedicated assistance of Martha Robbins, who typed the manuscript; Ali Soleymani, who offered advice and assistance with the computer programs used to draw the illustrations; Erin Whikehart, my daughter, who helped me design the cover; and Dr. Graeme Wilson, Chairman of the Department of Physiological Optics, The University of Alabama at Birmingham School of Optometry, who was gracious and considerate in allowing me to see this project to completion.

# Chapter 1

## Proteins

### Review of Proteins

Proteins (from the Greek *prōtos,* primary) are polymers of amino acids linked together by peptide bonds (Figure 1-1). These polymers arbitrarily are called *peptides* when their molecular weight is less than 10 kilodaltons (kd) (Figure 1-2A) and *proteins* when their molecular weight exceeds 10 kd (Figure 1-2B).* Proteins were first described by Berzelius in 1838 (Stryer, 1988).

As end products of genetic expression, proteins serve many vital functions in cells and tissues of biologic constituents from viruses to humans. Such roles include: mechanical support, control of growth and differentiation, catalysis, transport and storage, motion, nerve propagation, and immune protection. In the eye, proteins are known to support the structure and clarity of the cornea, to participate in the variable light refraction of the lens, to initiate the transduction of light into electrical signals, to generate intraocular pressure, and to lyse bacteria in the precorneal tear film. They have many other functions that indirectly sustain vision.

The amino acids that constitute proteins are molecules that contain at least one carboxyl and one amino group that is attached to the adjacent carbon (the alpha carbon) atom (Figure 1-3). Amino acids are distinguished from one another by the groups that are attached to the alpha carbon. It is reasonable to conclude that a protein is the sum of the functional properties of its constituent amino acids, but it is unreasonable to think that it is possible to accurately predict what properties they impart to an individual protein. Certain generalizations do apply, however. Twenty amino acids (Table 1-1) are commonly found in proteins, of which the dicarboxylic, diamino, amido, and hydroxy types contribute to the water solubility of a protein by their charged or polar nature. This is also true of amino acids positioned at the amino (N) and carboxyl (C) terminal ends of a protein. Cysteine also contributes to water solubility. All amino acids have in peptides and proteins their α-amino and associated carboxylate groups bound up in peptide bonds except at the N- and C-terminal ends (see Figure 1-2).

*A dalton (d) is a unit of mass close to that of hydrogen, which is 1.0000).

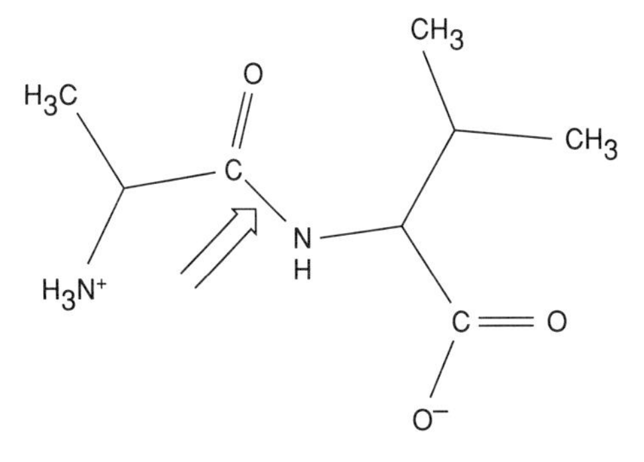

**FIGURE 1-1  The dipeptide alanylvaline.**
This peptide is made up of two amino acids linked by a peptide bond (*arrow*). Proteins consist of at least 80 amino acids joined by peptide bonds at their respective carboxylate and alpha amino groups.

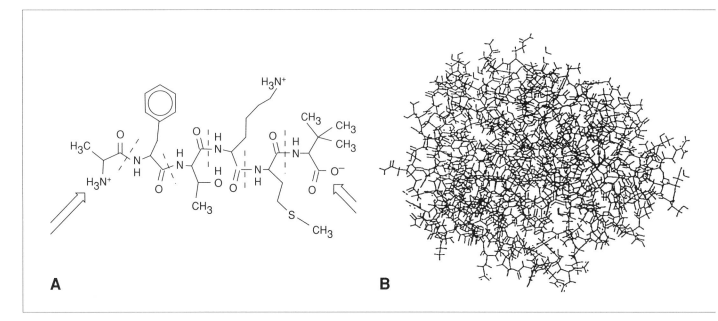

**FIGURE 1-2   (A) The peptide
ALA—PHE—THR—LYS—MET—LEU.**
This hexapeptide has five peptide bonds (*dotted lines*) and a molecular weight of 710 d. The N-terminal and C-terminal ends are indicated by arrows. The minimal complexity of a protein may be imagined by considering a molecule 14 times this large. (*B*) The protein elastase. From the Protein Data Bank, Brookhaven National Laboratory, Upton, NY.

Aromatic and unsubstituted amino acids, methionine, and proline impart hydrophobic (i.e., lipid-soluble) properties to proteins. These characteristics are important in the determination of conformational shapes, subunit binding (i.e., the association of more than one polypeptide chain), reactive site formation and function, as well as the existence of some proteins in cell membranes. Still other amino acids are involved in specialized functions that promote metal chelation (as histidine does in hemoglobin), chain binding (as cysteine does in the enzyme ribonuclease), and tight helical turns (as glycine does in collagen). All of these characteristics are significant, to greater or lesser degrees, for the function of each protein and these characteristics are dependent on where and how often each particular amino acid occurs in sequence (*primary structure*).

Proteins may be classified by several criteria: function, solubility, size, and biologic location are common ones. For example, using solubility as a factor, proteins are considered to be either water soluble (e.g., blood plasma proteins such as albumin), lipid soluble (e.g., intrinsic membrane proteins such as rhodopsin), or insoluble (e.g., extracellular matrix proteins such as collagen). Proteins are capable of being rendered nonfunctional by a process called *denaturation,* which can result from changes in temperature, ionic composition, or other environmental conditions. Denaturation alters at least some of the conformation of the protein from its native form. Denaturation can be temporary or permanent. Enzymes (catalytic proteins) are particularly prone to denaturation.

Contemporary understanding of proteins and their functions has been greatly aided by investigations of their genetic expression from deoxyribonucleic acid (DNA) and ribonucleic acid (RNA) as well as by studies of their structural representation via x-ray crystallography. Much more about the role of nucleic acids is included in Chapter 5. Crystallographic studies have yielded three-dimensional representations of proteins that may be exquisitely detailed with the aid of computer-driven molecular modeling (see Figures 1-2B and 1-4). Protein structure may be considered to fall into four basic divisions: primary, secondary, tertiary, and quaternary. As an example, let us consider the general structure of immunoglobulins (proteins

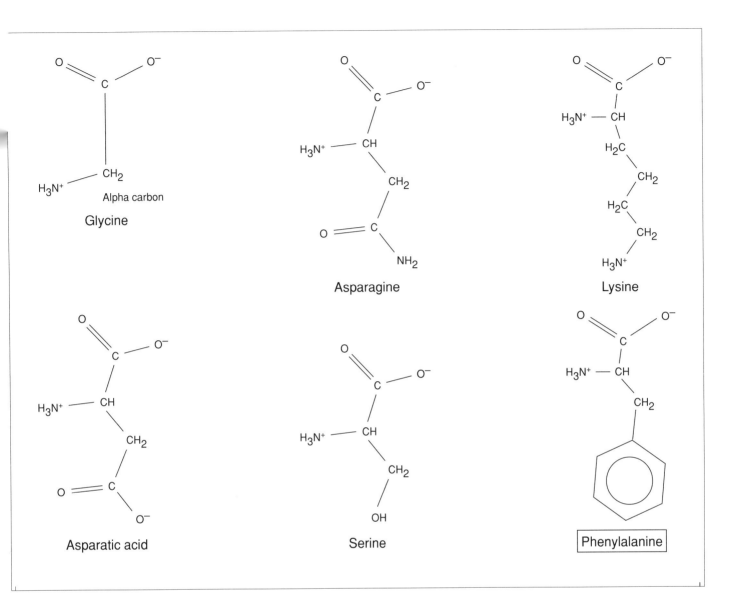

**FIGURE 1-3  Some representative amino acids.**
See Table 1-1 for the class to which each belongs and some of their properties. The actual charge characteristic of each amino acid in a protein may be determined by eliminating the charges on the carboxylate and alpha amino groups, except when they occur at the N- and C-terminals of a protein. Figure is continued on the next page.

involved in binding to antigens or foreign bodies such as bacteria). Typically immunoglobulins are composed of four polypeptide chains, each having its own particular sequence of amino acids.

The sequence of amino acids (named from left to right, starting at the free amino group or N-terminal end) is the *primary structure* of the protein (Figure 1-5). The immunoglobulins have at least four separate primary structures. Each sequence of amino acids is able to assume at least four different types of configurations or shapes due to the bulkiness, charge density, and hydrophobic regions of the amino acids in sequence. The shapes are further determined by hydrogen and disulfide bonding within and between amino acid chains.

Three types of *secondary structures* occur in immunoglobulins: *random coils, β-turns, and β-pleated sheets* (Figure 1-6). They make up part of the shape of one heavy chain. Another secondary structure present in proteins, but not in immunoglobulins, is the *α-helix* (discussed later). A structural or

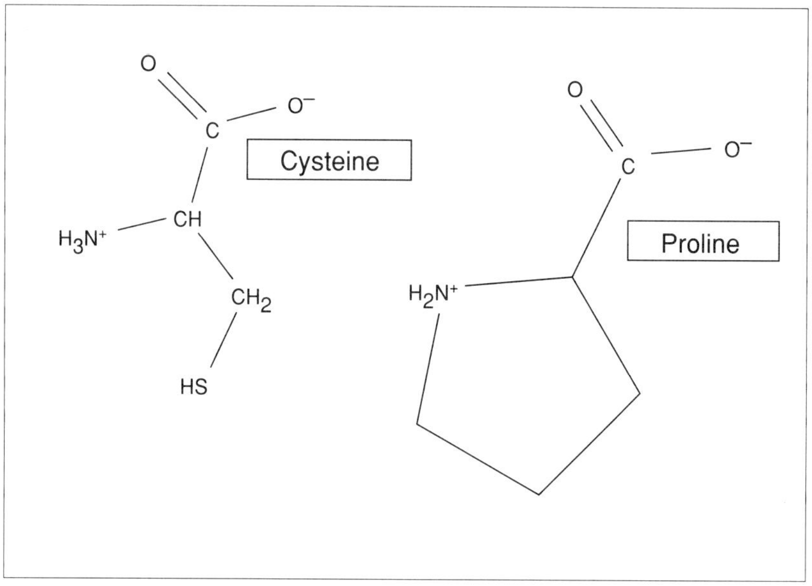

Cysteine

Proline

**FIGURE 1-3    (continued)**

functional part of one chain containing such structures has more recently been termed a *domain*, as shown in that same figure.

The entire shape of one polypeptide chain constitutes its *tertiary structure* (Figure 1-7). It can be seen that there are four globular masses, or domains, in the chain. These are the same domains as shown in Figure 1-6, except that they have been filled in. A domain may be considered, therefore, as either a subdivision of a tertiary structure or a discrete collection of secondary structures.

Finally, the *quaternary structure* of the immunoglobulin is the total conformation assumed by all the polypeptides that make up a protein. Figure 1-8 shows the shape assumed by the two light chains and the two heavy chains.

One other kind of secondary structure found in other proteins is a helix (Figure 1-9). Some helical structures may also be seen in the computer-drawn protein in Figure 1-4. There are several kinds of helices that can be found in specific proteins. It is worthwhile to mention, however, that α-helices are the most common ones in soluble proteins and in the portions of proteins that traverse membranes. Rhodopsin, for example, contains a considerable proportion of α-helical structure. On the other hand, β-pleated sheets dominate the lens-soluble proteins known as crystallins.

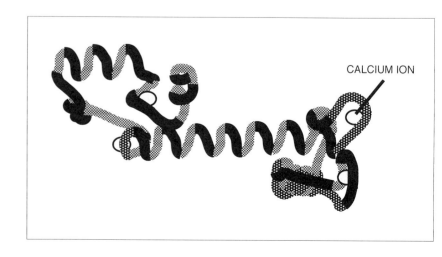

**FIGURE 1-4    Redrawn model of calmodulin, a protein that stores calcium ions inside cells.**
The location of four calcium ions is evident, as is the extensive helical structure of the protein. Adapted from Babu YS, Bugg CE, and Cook WJ. Structure of calmodulin. *In Molecular Aspects of Cellular Regulation. V. Calmodulin.* Cohen P, and Klee CB, eds. Amsterdam: Elsevier, 1988.

**TABLE 1-1  Amino Acids Found in Proteins and Peptides**

| Type | Name | Abbreviations | Remarks |
|---|---|---|---|
| Unsubstituted | Glycine* <br> Alanine <br> Valine <br> Leucine <br> Isoleucine | Gly/G <br> Ala/A <br> Val/V <br> Leu/L <br> Ile/I | Impart hydrophobic characteristics to proteins. Glycine can give a tighter "twist" to proteins such as collagen. |
| Dicarboxylic | Aspartic*† <br> Glutamic† | Asp/D <br> Glu/E | Impart negative charges to proteins due to ionization of one carboxylate |
| Diamino | Lysine* <br> Arginine <br> Histidine | Lys/K <br> Arg/R <br> His/H | Impart positive charges to proteins due to ionization of one amine |
| Amido | Asparagine* <br> Glutamine | Asn/N <br> Glu/Q | Derived from Asp and Glu, they are hydrophilic. |
| Hydroxy | Serine* <br> Threonine | Ser/S <br> Thr/T | Hydroxy groups render them hydrophilic. |
| Aromatic | Phenylalanine* <br> Tyrosine <br> Tryptophan | Phe/F <br> Tyr/Y <br> Trp/W | Impart hydrophobic characteristics to proteins. Tyrosine is less hydrophobic due to its OH group. |
| Sulfur | Cysteine* <br><br> Methionine | Cys/C <br><br> Met/M | Cys forms disulfide bonds between peptide chains and imparts hydrophilic characteristics. Met imparts hydrophobic characteristics. |
| Cyclic | Proline* | Pro/P | Nonaromatic, Pro is found in insoluble extracellular collagen, elastin, and mucin. |

*Structure shown in Figure 1-3.

†Also called aspartate and glutamate, to represent their ionized forms.

There are also several variations of β-pleated sheet structure. Both α-helices and β-pleated sheets are stabilized by hydrogen bonds. These are weak bonds that form between hydrogen and either oxygen or nitrogen. They occur as a result of the electron-withdrawing properties of other oxygen

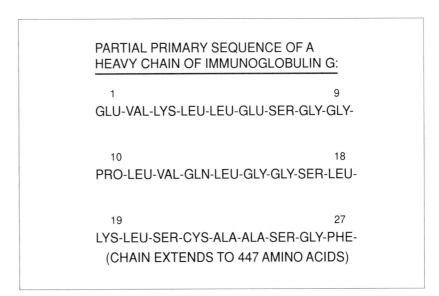

**PARTIAL PRIMARY SEQUENCE OF A HEAVY CHAIN OF IMMUNOGLOBULIN G:**

1                                                              9
GLU-VAL-LYS-LEU-LEU-GLU-SER-GLY-GLY-

10                                                            18
PRO-LEU-VAL-GLN-LEU-GLY-GLY-SER-LEU-

19                                                            27
LYS-LEU-SER-CYS-ALA-ALA-SER-GLY-PHE-
(CHAIN EXTENDS TO 447 AMINO ACIDS)

**FIGURE 1-5  Primary protein structure.**
The structure consists of the sequence of amino acids beginning at the N-terminal end of each polypeptide chain in the protein.

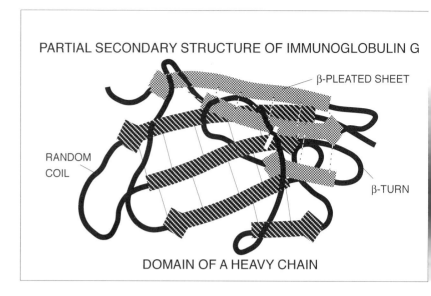

**FIGURE 1-6   Secondary protein structure within a sequence of amino acids.**
Four types are generally recognized: helices, pleated sheets, random coils, and turns. Three are shown here. A domain is a collection of secondary structures that have some functional importance. Hydrogen bonds are shown by thin lines. One disulfide bond is represented by a thick white line.

and nitrogen atoms and give the hydrogen atom a partial positive charge. Proteins vary enormously in molecular weight, from 10 kd to several million daltons. Table 1-2 lists some representative proteins. Many proteins that contain more than one polypeptide chain are held together by sulfur bridges known as *disulfide bonds*. The four chains of immunoglobulin G (IgG) (see Figure 1-8) are joined in this manner. Some proteins have their peptide chains altered after synthesis. The process is called: *posttranslational modification.*

In addition to their specialized functions, proteins may act as reservoirs of positive and negative charges and, therefore, constitute intracellular or extracellular pH buffers. In general, negative charges tend to predominate in proteins at the physiological pH of blood serum (7.4), which may vary from intracellular pH values. Proteins are an important source for the generation of osmotic pressure across cell boundaries. This is a significant function in the eye with respect to processes such as corneal deturgescence (the mechanism in which the corneal stroma is maintained in a clear state) and the generation of intraocular pressure (which contributes to ocular viscoelasticity). The discussion that follows considers five significant proteins found in ocular tissues.

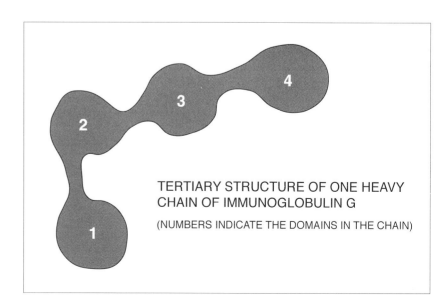

**FIGURE 1-7   Tertiary protein structure.**
This structure represents the entire conformation assumed by one polypeptide chain, but several domains may be contained within its overall shape.

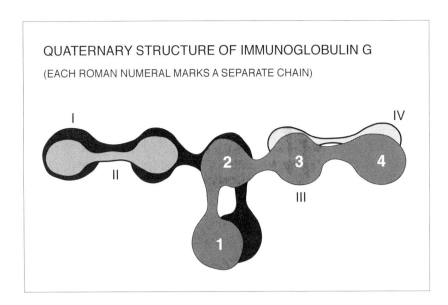

**FIGURE 1-8 Quaternary protein structure.**
This is the entire conformation of a protein that consists of two or more polypeptide chains. Single polypeptide chain proteins have no quaternary structure.

## Crystallins

### Characteristics

The crystallins are a family of proteins found in the epithelial and fiber cells of the ocular lens. They are water-soluble proteins whose major classification was originally based on their relative ability to migrate in an electric field (i.e., electrophoresis). They were identified as α-, β-, and γ-crystallins. However, β-crystallins can be further divided into $\beta_H$ (heavy) and $\beta_L$ (light) groups. Although this classification remains, numerous members of each group now are known, and this has been a source of confusion even among

**TABLE 1-2 Molecular Weight of Some Proteins**

| Protein | Approximate Molecular Weight in Daltons | Function |
|---|---|---|
| Lysozyme | 14,000 | Enzyme (catalyst) in tears that lyses the peptidoglycan in cell walls of Gram-positive bacteria. |
| γ-Crystallin | 20,000 | Soluble protein in lens fiber cells that contributes to the lens structure |
| Rhodopsin | 40,000 | Integral membrane protein of rod outer segments that mediates visual transduction. |
| Hemoglobin: | | Protein that carries oxygen to tissues. |
| Two α units each each at | 16,000 | |
| Two β units each at | 16,000 | |
| Total | 64,000 | |
| $Na^+K^+$ATPase: | | Integral membrane enzyme that pumps sodium out of cells while pumping potassium inward. |
| Two α units each at | 112,000 | |
| Two β units each at | 40,000 | |
| Total | 304,000 | |
| Tropocollagen (type I) | 400,000 | Single unit of collagen structure found in corneal stroma and in many other tissues. |
| Fibronectin: | | Connects cells with collagen. |
| Two units each at | 250,000 | |
| Total | 500,000 | |
| Laminin: | | Connects cells with basement membrane. |
| Three units each at | 330,000 | |
| Total | 990,000 | |
| HM crystallin (numerous units) | >5,000,000 | Aggregate in lens cells whose function is unknown. It may be a precataractous form. |

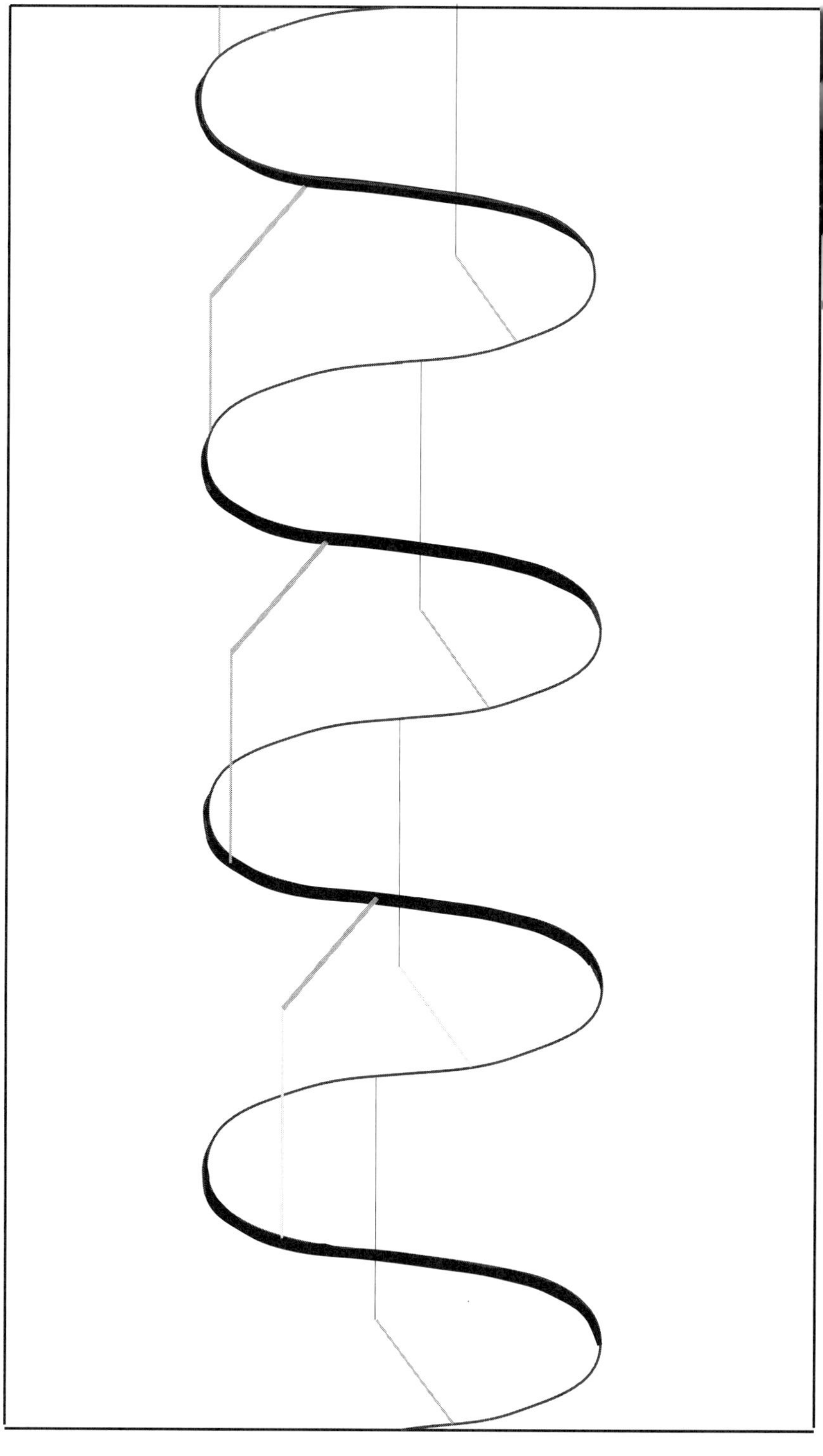

**FIGURE 1-9  Helical structure.**
This fourth type of secondary structure is usually an α-helix in most cellular proteins. An α-helix is defined as one that has a 1.5Å rise for every 100 degrees of rotation. Rhodopsin is an ocular protein with α-helical structure where it crosses disc membranes. Hydrogen bonds are shown as thin lines.

lens protein chemists. Although crystallins have been considered to be proteins unique to the eye, Wistow and Piatigorsky (1988) have hypothesized that the α-crystallins are related in origin to heat-shock proteins and to a schistosome (parasitic flatworm) egg antigen protein, whereas β- and γ-crystallins are related to a bacterial spore coat protein that binds calcium. More recently, as reviewed by Horwitz (1993), it was found that α-crystallins also occur in nonocular tissues such as heart, brain, and lung. Other crystallin types are known, but they are not found in adult humans.

The role of these proteins, though they are water soluble, has been termed *structural* (Harding and Crabbe, 1984). This means that they serve to maintain the elongated shape of lens fiber cells and, ultimately, the lens structure itself. This is emphasized by the fact that the average concentration of lens proteins is about twice that of most other intracellular proteins (33% versus 15%). In other words, the packing or high concentration of such proteins helps to maintain lens shape. The medical and scientific interest in crystallins has been dominated by their possible involvement in senile cataract formation. An examination of their chemical and physical characteristics is helpful in understanding their constitution (Table 1-3).

The primary structures (sequences) of α- and β-crystallins are altered by a number of cellular biochemical reactions. Acetylation (the addition of acetyl groups at the N-terminus) is a mechanism that prevents the cellular

TABLE 1-3  Characteristics of Mammalian Crystallins

| Properties | Crystallin | | |
| --- | --- | --- | --- |
| | α | β | γ |
| Primary structure | N-terminal acetylated; sequence varies and is modified.* | N-terminal acetylated and modified* | N-terminal glycine; sequence is unique and is not modified |
| Secondary structure | α-Helical and β-pleated[†] sheets | β-pleated[†] sheets | β-pleated sheets[†] |
| Tertiary structure | Probably globular | Probably globular | Globular |
| Quaternary structure | Large globe of four different polypeptides (20 kd each) | Large globe of polypeptides of 23.5–35 kd | None; it has a single polypeptide. |
| Molecular weight (kd) | 800 | 50 ($\beta_L$) 160 ($\beta_H$) | 20 |
| Cysteine content (residues) | 107* | 11 ($\beta_L$)[‡] 33 ($\beta_H$) | 6[§] |
| pI [∥] | ~4.9 | ~6.4 | ~7.6 |
| Relative proportion (%)[¶] | ~35 | ~55 | ~10 |

*Proteins undergo posttranslational modification (i.e., they are modified after they are synthesized).

[†]See Figure 1-10. Recent studies suggest that α-crystallins have predominantly α-helical structure (Farnsworth et al., 1993).

[‡]Data recalculated from Spector (1984), as residues per 1000 residues using molecular weights and an average amino acid molecular weight of 120.

[§]Data recalculated from Summers et al. (1986) for human γ 1-2 crystallin, as residues per 1000 residues using molecular weights and an average amino acid molecular weight of 120.

[∥] The isoelectric point (pI) is the pH at which the number of positive and negative charges on a protein are equal. The pI indicates the charge characteristics of a specific protein and can be used to separate proteins. Values are approximate due to the existence of more than one component for each type.

[¶]Values are for whole lens. Exact percentages vary from species to species. Alpha-crystallin is the only crystallin type in lens epithelium. All three types occur in lens fiber cells (see Harding, 1981).

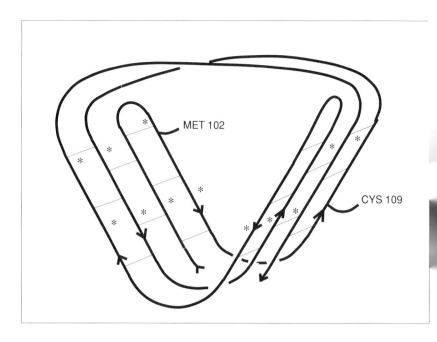

**FIGURE 1-10  A domain of γ-crystallin (approximately half the molecule).**
A domain is a portion of a protein that may contain one or more secondary structures. Here are seen two β-pleated sheets formed in a V with hydrogen bonds (*thin lines*) connecting the polypeptide chains. There are two wide random turns at the top of the structure. Each asterisk indicates the presence of a hydrophobic amino acid. Methionine (No. 102) and cysteine (No. 109) are potential sites of oxidation of the protein. Oxidation can promote crystallin aggregation. (Summers et al., 1986)

degradation of a protein. This means that the α- and β-crystallins, once synthesized, are quite stable. The primary structures of α- and β-crystallins are nonetheless altered after synthesis by the addition of phosphate groups (phosphorylation), the incorporation of sugars (glycosylation), or the possible removal of amide groups (deamidation). Phosphorylation increases the negative charges and potential energy of a protein. Glycosylation, a common characteristic of many proteins, does not seem to have been assigned a role in crystallins. Deamidation may be an artifact of crystallin preparation, although some investigators have identified it as part of the lens aging process.

The secondary structure of all human crystallins is characterized by the existence of β-pleated sheets (Figure 1-10), though α-crystallins may have considerable helical structure (Farnsworth et al., 1993). This protein substructure consists of rows of the same polypeptide chain that runs antiparallel and is held together by hydrogen bonds (the thin lines in the figure). β-pleated sheets can incorporate a number of hydrophobic amino acids (asterisks in the figure). In the case of the γ-crystallins, two sets of these sheets (called *motifs*) are aligned in a V shape to form a hydrophobic globular structure known as a *domain* (as previously mentioned for immunoglobulins). Each γ-crystallin (tertiary structure) contains two domains, which, though considerably hydrophobic, are still remarkably water soluble! This means that they are still water soluble on their surface but are lipid soluble in their interior.

The β-crystallins are thought to have a similar conformation. These secondary structures, therefore, determine the globular nature of the three crystallins (i.e., its tertiary structure). The α-crystallins, although incorporating β-pleated sheets, have not yet had their structures adequately described. However, they may also be globular. The structures are potentially important in determining lens fiber cell architecture.

The quaternary structure of α- and β-crystallins is often simply called an *aggregate*. This means that the final shape is determined by the binding of more than one kind of polypeptide chain. In the case of α-crystallins, four separate polypeptide chains have been described from bovine lens: A1, A2, B1, and B2. They are assembled in undefined combinations of the four kinds of chains. A2 and B2 are the primary gene products having separate amino acid sequences, whereas A1 and B1 are modifications of A2 and B2 after sequencing (Harding and Crabbe, 1984). Some of these modifications involve phosphorylation of the polypeptides. Chiesa et al. (1989) found that phosphorylation of the A2 chain (to A1) was maximal in mature lens fiber cells and that phosphorylation of the B2 chain (to B1) became minimal in mature lens fiber cells. In general, the total amount of phosphorylation of the chains of $\alpha$-crystallin is increased as lens fiber cells mature. However, a correlation of these changes with exact cell function has not been made. Horwitz (1993) has described $\alpha$-crystallins as being protective as well as structural. They seem to prevent the structural denaturation of all lens proteins, a phenomenon known as a *chaperone function.*

The number of separate polypeptides in $\beta$-crystallins is larger than that of the other crystallins. Broadly, the chains are divided into two groups: $\beta_H$ (molecular weight $\sim$160 kd) and $\beta_L$ (molecular weight $\sim$50 kd). More recent studies suggest that there are two $\beta_L$ fractions as well as a $\beta_S$ (s = single chain) fraction (the latter being a monomer).[1] Berbers et al. (1982) identified six different polypeptides as members of the $\beta$-crystallin family that are the primary gene products. Post-translational modifications further augment this number of polypeptides in $\beta$-crystallin aggregates. The exact compositions of these aggregates remain unknown. Life is indeed complicated for the lens protein chemist.

The cysteine content of the various crystallins is important inasmuch as each cysteine group is a potential source of molecular bridging or aggregation via disulfide bonding. Such aggregation is discussed in more detail in the section on cataract formation. In Table 1-3, under Cysteine content, the numbers refer to the cysteine atoms per protein molecule. The $\alpha$-crystallins, on this basis, would seem to have the greatest potential for aggregation by disulfide bonding. Indeed, $\alpha$-crystallins form the highest–molecular weight aggregates under normal conditions. This is somewhat offset by its chaperone function of maintaining normal conformation without aggregation. However, there exist even higher–molecular weight aggregates in cataractous lenses that contain all three crystallin types. Cysteine content, therefore, is a relative criterion for aggregation. The isoelectric point (pI, the pH at which the sum of positive and negative charges in a protein are equal) of each crystallin indicates that $\alpha$-crystallin is the most acidic. This is so since it has the most negative charges at physiological pH (7.4). Gamma-crystallin, in contrast, has the fewest negative charges at physiological pH. The significance of these pI values, besides showing a charge variation of the proteins, seems to point to a relatively open or spread-out conformation of the $\alpha$-crystallins, particularly those that have been phosphorylated in mature lens fiber cells.

The crystallins account for about 90% of all soluble lens proteins. The relative proportions of the crystallins in the lens are: $\alpha$-crystallins, 35%; $\beta$-crystallins, 55%; and $\gamma$-crystallins, 10% (Bours and Hockwin, 1976). It should be noted that $\alpha$-crystallins are the only crystallins found in the lens epithelium. Consequently, $\beta$- and $\gamma$-crystallins are characteristic of lens fiber cells, though $\alpha$-crystallins also occur there.

## Cataract Formation

The formation of senile cataracts has been under investigation by crystallin protein chemists for many years, but significant progress has been made

---

[1]Some investigators consider $\beta_S$ crystallin to be a member of the $\gamma$-crystallin family.

only in the past 20 years. Observations about crystallins in the normal aging lens to some degree parallel those observations made on crystallins in the cataractous lens.

The most general effect is the change in the amounts of soluble and insoluble lens proteins (Figure 1-11). The obvious difference between normal and cataractous lens proteins (of which the majority are crystallins) is the increased concentration of insoluble proteins and the associated decreased concentration of soluble proteins in the cataractous lens after about age 50 years (Spector, 1984). In the normal aging process, crystallins of the three major types become incorporated to some degree into the insoluble fraction of lens proteins, presumably by disulfide bonding of their cysteine amino acids as well as by other cross-linking. Of the insoluble proteins, only about 1% are the normally insoluble proteins of the cell plasma membranes. However, with advancing age this insoluble fraction accounts for 50% or more of all the lens protein.

It is known that several high–molecular weight aggregates (HM) of crystallins can be isolated from the human lens with advancing age. These are: HM1, HM2, HM3, and HM4. HM1 and HM2, with molecular weights in excess of one million daltons, are soluble crystallin complexes. Although evidence suggests that these fractions may be artifacts of preparation

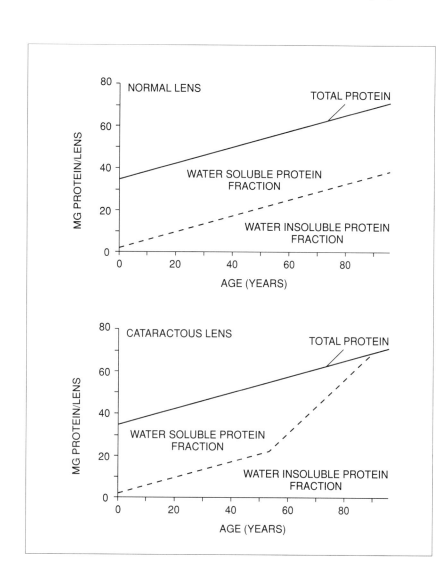

**FIGURE 1-11   Graphs of protein concentrations in (A) normal and (B) cataractous lenses.**
The areas between the lines represent the amounts of soluble and insoluble protein, respectively; the top line indicates total protein. (Adapted from Spector, 1984).

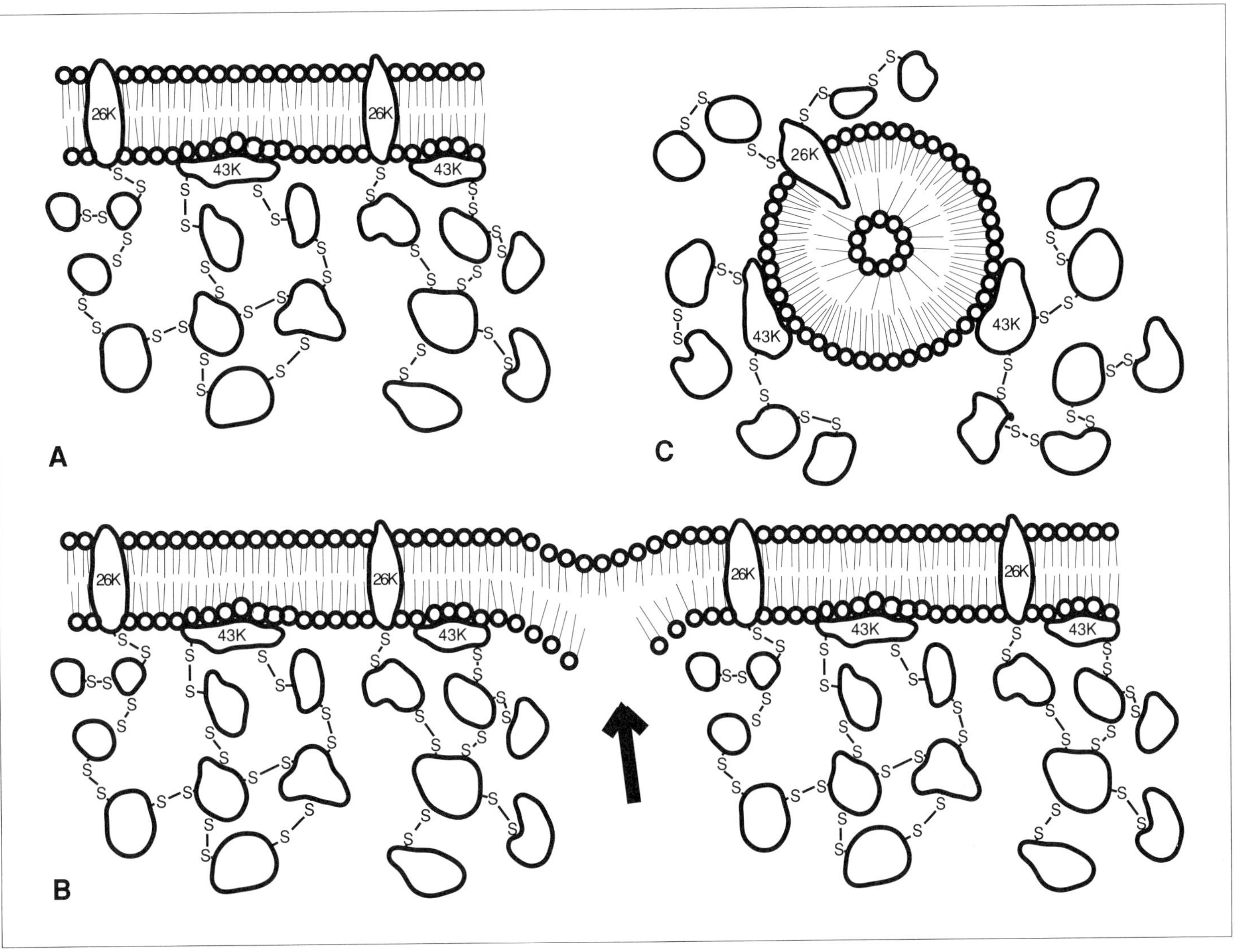

**FIGURE 1-12   The proposed aggregation of lens proteins in senile cataract formation.**

Both nuclear and cortical cataracts form aggregates (*A*). The aggregrated crystallins (*white blobs*) are seen bound to each other by disulfide (or other) bonds. They are also bound to 43 kd and 26 kd proteins at the plasma membrane of the lens fiber cells. In cortical cataracts the aggregation proceeds to cause a rupture in the membrane (*B, arrow*), which destroys lens fiber cells and produces cellular debris (*C*). (Adapted from Spector, 1984).

(Harding and Crabbe, 1984), they nonetheless occur more often in older lenses and in more mature (i.e., interior) sections of lenses at all ages.

The HM3 and HM4 aggregates are found only in cataractous lenses. HM3 is insoluble and requires a strong denaturing agent such as guanidinium chloride for solubilization. This agent promotes unfolding and dissociation of the aggregate. HM3 is composed of a mixture of crystallins as well as a non-crystallin 43 kd protein located on the inner face of the plasma membranes of lens fiber cells. Spector (1984) has suggested that a 26 kd intrinsic membrane protein may also be part of the HM fractions that occur in cataracts. HM3 has a molecular weight range between 2 and $33 \times 10^6$, a very large molecular species (Harding and Crabbe, 1984). HM3 is held together by disulfide bonds and is associated with cortical cataracts. Fraction HM4 is composed of cross-links that are not disulfide bonded and occurs exclusively in nuclear cataracts. HM4 is also insoluble and requires a denaturing agent for solubilization. This fraction is associated with the dark color of nuclear cataracts, but the source of the color is speculative (Harding, 1981). It is an important observation that the color of fraction HM4 causes a cataract to absorb light as well as to scatter it (Lerman and Borkman, 1976). This double-barrelled component of nuclear cataract formation increases the severity of visual impairment. The properties of these HM fractions are summarized in Table 1-4.

**TABLE 1-4  Properties of HM Aggregates of Crystallins**

| Fraction | Composition | Molecular Weight ($10^6$ d) | Solubility | Occurrence |
|---|---|---|---|---|
| HM1* | α-crystallin | >1 | Soluble | All lenses |
| HM2* | α-, β-, γ-crystallins | >1 | Soluble | All lenses |
| HM3* | α-, β-, γ-crystallins‡, 43 kd protein | 2–33 | Insoluble | Cataractous (cortical lenses) |
| HM4 | α-, β-, γ-crystallins‡, 43 kd protein | >5 | Insoluble | Cataractous (nuclear lenses) |

*Disulfide linked.

†Not disulfide linked but contains one or more light-absorbing (i.e., colored) components.

‡May also bond to a 26 kd protein.

It has been hypothesized that senile cataracts develop as a result of growing HM fractions, which form at the inner layer of the lens cell plasma membranes and grow into the cell cytoplasm. The protein complexes continue to grow as the lens ages by forming either disulfide bonds or other covalent bonds (Figure 1-12A). Both cortical and nuclear cataracts start out as at "A" in the figure, although nuclear cataracts have different cross-links. This is the stage to which nuclear cataracts form. However, an important difference with cortical cataracts, is that the strain produced in the cell membrane by the growing HM aggregates (see Figure 1-12B) leads to membrane rupture (*arrow*). The resultant cellular debris would include membrane fragments such as the micellar form (Figure 1-12C), to which are attached HM crystallin aggregates. These would, at least partially, constitute the fragmented or globular formations that are described clinically.

The reason that such an aggregation of disulfide-bonded and other cross-linked crystallins occurs is not certain. Nor is it certain how great the aggregations must be before they cause membrane disruption. Some older patients have limited lens fiber cell disruption and yet have clinically clear lenses. In the case of disulfide-bonded crystallins, Garner and Spector (1980) have shown that the oxidation state of both methionine and cysteine in the crystallins and in the 43 kd protein of normal (60- to 65-year-old) human lenses is different from that of cataractous lenses of the same age. These investigators suggested that in the normal state the sulfur-containing amino acids are buried in a normal protein conformation and are prevented from oxidizing (i.e., forming both sulfoxide and disulfide bonds). Minimal oxidation of exposed groups, however, may cause conformational changes in the crystallins that eventually expose other groups, which in turn oxidize and bring about aggregate formation. Glutathione (a tripeptide: γGLU—CYS—GLY) is thought to protect crystallins from cross-linking by binding to such exposed groups. However, evidence indicates that the function of glutathione is overwhelmed in cataract formation (Spector, 1984). This cross-linking would apply only to cortical aggregates that form cortical cataracts (Figure 1-13). The process of progressive oxidation might be introduced by extralenticular hydrogen peroxide in the aqueous (Spector, 1984).

The cause of nuclear cataracts is more obscure, and the nature of the color in brunescent nuclear cataracts remains speculative. The tryptophan amino acid components of crystallins have been suspected to be the cause (Harding and Crabbe, 1984). Normally, there is an increase in yellow coloration of the lens which augments with age and which had been thought to be associated with tryptophan changes. Radiation in the range of 300 to 400 nm (including sunlight) has the potential of being cataractogenic, since the lens absorbs these wavelengths. A possible connection between such ultraviolet light and tryptophan alteration was suggested by Pirie (1971, 1972), who reported that ultraviolet light was able to oxidize tryptophan to synurenine kynurenine in proteins in vitro (Figure 1-14 A, B). She thought that such altered amino acids in crystallins may lead to the brown color of nuclear cataracts. It was also indicated that this process might eventually lead to the nondisulfide cross-linking that is characteristic of HM4 aggregates found in nuclear cataracts. Dilley and Pirie (1974) later reported that the loss of tryptophan observed in vitro did not occur in brown cataracts and that the yellowing coloration, associated with aging, progresses equally in the cortical as well as the nuclear regions of a human lens. The suggestion here is that yellowing of the lens may be a separate event from the formation of a brown cataract, which occurs only in the nucleus. Other investigators have argued that either (1) damaging free radicals (unpaired electrons) are produced from tryptophan (Weiter and Finch, 1975) or (2) only a minimal number of tryptophan residues need to be destroyed to bring about cataractogenesis (Lerman and Borkman, 1976). Very little evidence has come forth to support these arguments, however, and so the hypothesis of a possible connection between ultraviolet radiation, tryptophan alteration in crystallins, and brown coloration of the lens nucleus is largely unproven.

Possibly apart from the issue of ultraviolet sunlight, but still implicating tryptophan, Dillon et al. (1976) observed β-carboline products in normal and cataractous lenses, and Truscott (1977) and Garcia-Castineiras, et al. (1978), respectively observed anthranilic acid (anthranilate) in cataractous

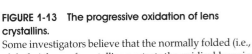

**FIGURE 1-13   The progressive oxidation of lens crystallins.**

Some investigators believe that the normally folded (i.e., globular) form of crystallins protects the oxidizable amino acids methionine (—S—CH$_3$) and cysteine (—SH) (A). In the course of aggregation, methionine is first oxidized to —SO—CH$_3$, possibly by hydrogen peroxide in the adjacent aqueous. This action could partially unfold the protein (B). Subsequently, the exposed cysteines would oxidize, as —S—S—, forming disulfide bonds with other crystallins and membrane proteins in a series of chain reactions, as at C and D.

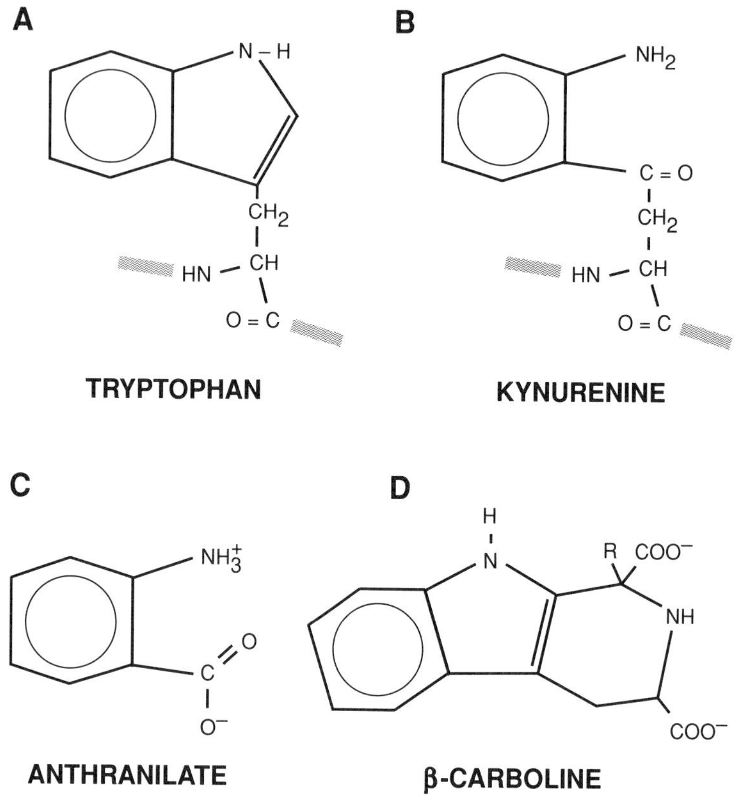

FIGURE 1-14  The oxidation of the amino acid tryptophan to kynurenine can be obtained in proteins in vitro by ultraviolet light (as in *A* and *B*). However, no relationship has been established between the possible formation of kynurenine in the lens and any coloration of the lens. Anthranilate, a breakdown product of kynurenine (in C) has been found in cataractous lenses. Beta-carboline, an example of one of many forms, is shown in *D*. It has also been found in the lens and the compound may represent a fused ring form of tryptophan and another amino acid in crystallins that produce yellow or brown coloration.

lenses. It has been suggested that β-carbolines may represent the nondisulfide cross-link structures of tryptophan with another amino acid in crystallins. Anthranilate may be a breakdown product of tryptophan found in crystallins of nuclear cataracts (Figure 1-14C, D).

## Rhodopsin and Cone Pigment Proteins

There was a time when virtually all ocular biochemistry was centered on the subject of rhodopsin. This was the case since rhodopsin is at the heart of the process of *visual transduction:* the conversion of light energy into electrical signalling that the brain interprets as sight. It is now known that a much more complex process is involved in visual transduction and that rhodopsin only initiates that process. Here, the focus will be on rhodopsin and cone pigment proteins per se. In Chapter 6 the connection of rhodopsin with visual transduction is described in detail. Rhodopsin is a protein that was first described by the German scientist Franz Boll in 1876 as a red-purple visual pigment. Afterwards, Willy Kühne (a contemporary of Boll) described the pigment as "regenerable" in a light-dark cycle. He extracted the pigment from the retina and first described its spectral properties. In more recent times, the American scientist George Wald showed the relationship of vitamin A to rhodopsin (Bridges, 1970).

*Rhodopsin* is an intrinsic membrane protein found in the discs, and to a lesser extent in the plasma membranes, of the rod outer segments of photoreceptor cells in the retina. As an intrinsic membrane protein, its structure extends completely through the disc membrane (Figure 1-15). Like many membrane proteins, rhodopsin is best made analogous to a boat floating in a sea of phospholipids and other lipids that constitute the discs as well as the plasma membranes of the rod photoreceptor. There are some constraints to this floating, however. The protein is always oriented in such a way that its N-terminal end is facing either the intradiscal space on the disc membrane or the interphotoreceptor matrix (extracellular space between photoreceptors) on the plasma membrane. This is indicated by the taillike appendage on each rhodopsin molecule in Figure 1-15. This orientation is necessary so that the protein can maintain its functional role. Rhodopsin molecules are further constrained from migrating around the ends of the discs by a large, high–molecular weight protein present at the apex of each disc. This would seem to control the population of rhodopsin molecules on each side of the disc.

Rhodopsin has a molecular weight of approximately 41 kd and has conformational features as shown in Figure 1-16. The N-terminal region has two short-chain sugars (carbohydrates), which anchor or orient the molecule. The C-terminal region contains several hydroxy amino acids, which can be phosphorylated (as indicated by P's). Phosphorylation seems to act

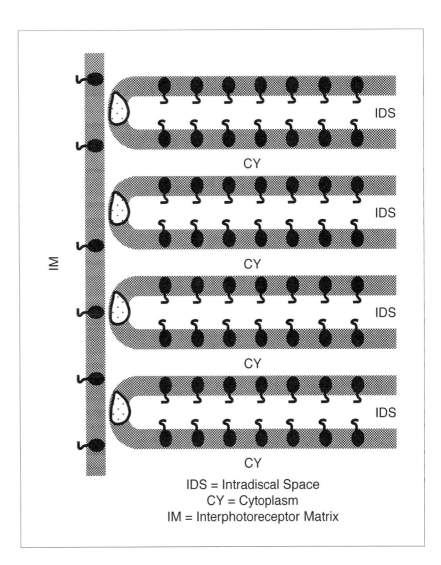

**FIGURE 1-15 Diagram of a cross section of a rod outer segment showing the placement of rhodopsin molecules (*black ovals with hooks*) in the discs and plasma membrane of the rod.**
The hooks represent sugar-containing N-termini of the molecules that prevent molecular flip-flopping and maintain the orientation of the molecules. It is well known that the vast majority of rhodopsin molecules are in the discs. A large membrane protein located at each end of the disc (speckled oval) prevents rhodopsin from migrating around the ends of the discs. (Adapted from Anderson RE. *Biochemistry of the Eye.* San Francisco: American Academy of Ophthalmology, 1983;169.)

IDS = Intradiscal Space
CY = Cytoplasm
IM = Interphotoreceptor Matrix

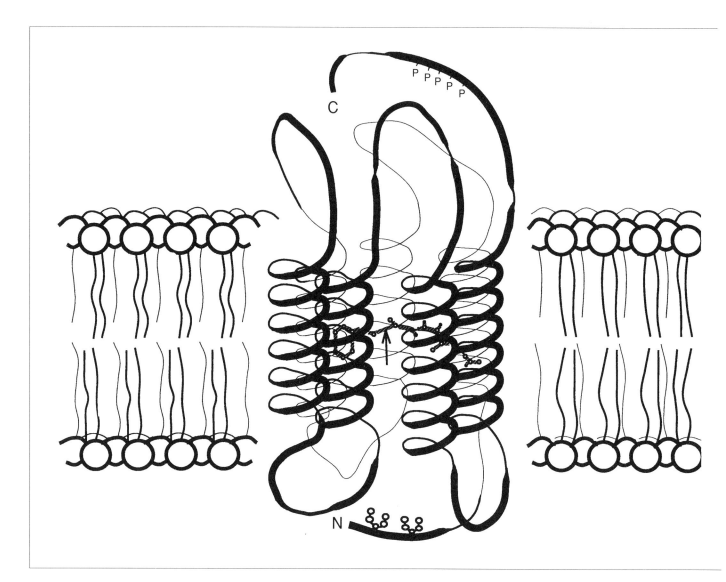

**FIGURE 1-16  Representation of a rhodopsin molecule situated in a rod disc membrane.**

Note the seven α-helices in the area of the membrane, the 11-*cis* retinal buried within the helices (*arrow*), the small sugar chains at the N-terminus (*small spheres*), and the phosphorylated serine amino acids near the C-terminus (where the phosphate groups are located). (Adapted from Dratz EA, and Hargrave PA. *Trends Biochem Sci* 1983;8:128.)

as a mechanism for "fine tuning" the sensitivity of the protein to light. The portion of the molecule that traverses the membrane consists of seven α-helices (secondary structure), whose sequences (primary structure) are composed of substantial amounts of hydrophobic amino acids. This characteristic, common to many intrinsic membrane proteins, imparts a strong association of the protein with the lipids that make up the disc membrane.

Rhodopsin has an additional, nonprotein component, vitamin A, which is contained within the membrane-associated portion of the molecule (Figure 1-16, *arrow*). This component or moiety is present as the aldehyde form and is most simply known as *retinal*. The vitamin is bound to the protein at the amino acid lysine, No. 296 from the N-terminal end of the molecule. As part of the rhodopsin molecule, the conformation of retinal is in the 11-*cis* form (Figure 1-17), which represents the most energetically favorable configuration for its confinement among the helices of the protein. The bond linkage of the aldehyde form with the protein is that of a protonated (H+ added) Schiff base:

$$Retinal—CH = NH^+—Opsin \qquad (1\text{-}1)$$

**FIGURE 1-17** Conversion of rhodopsin to all-*trans* retinal and opsin.

hodopsin is shown at the top as 11-*cis* retinal bound to psin via a protonated Schiff base. The initial reaction (*1*), aused by a photon of light striking the molecule, is the onversion of 11-*cis* retinal to all-*trans* retinal while bound to the protein producing bathorhodopsin (a form in which he structure of retinal is strained). Three intermediate orms are then rapidly made in sequence (*2*): umirhodopsin, metarhodopsin I, and metarhodopsin II the last form shown). Each of these forms, having its own pectral properties, produces slightly different protein onformations, which are not shown. In the conversion of metarhodopsin I to metarhodopsin II the Schiff base is eprotonated. Metarhodopsin II, also known as *photoexcited rhodopsin*, is discussed further in Chapter 6. Finally, the chiff base is broken (*3*) with the release of *all*-trans retinal nd opsin. Rhodopsin is regenerated in two stages (*4,5*). ll-*trans* retinal is isomerized to 11-*cis* retinal by the enzyme etinal isomerase (*4*), and the 11-*cis* retinal recombines with psin (*5*).

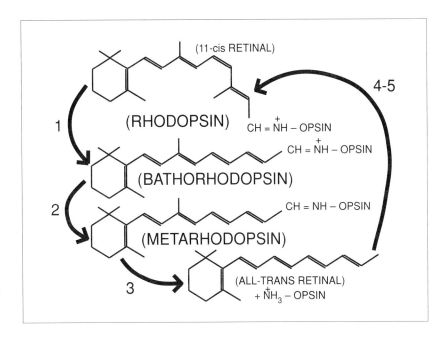

A Schiff base has the characteristic of being less permanent, or stable, than many covalent bonds, so vitamin A can be more easily detached from the protein by light stimulation.

Rhodopsin is referred to as a *holoprotein* when retinal is attached to lysine No. 296. In 1958 George Wald (1968) demonstrated that light isomerizes the 11-*cis* retinal group of rhodopsin to all-*trans* retinal (Figure 1-17). This creates an energetically unstable molecule that rapidly proceeds through several intermediate forms (bathorhodopsin, lumirhodopsin, metarhodopsin I and II) in which the Schiff base linkage is deprotonated, and finally broken (see Figure 1-17). The completion of the reaction results in the release of vitamin A (as all-*trans* retinal) from the protein. The protein then is called *opsin*. When any nonprotein portion of a holoprotein such as rhodopsin is released, the protein portion is labelled an *apoprotein*. Opsin is, therefore, an apoprotein. The nonprotein portion (such as vitamin A) represents a *prosthetic group*. Table 1-5 summarizes the properties of rhodopsin.

**TABLE 1-5  Properties of Rhodopsin**

| | |
|---|---|
| Molecular weight (d) | |
| Holoprotein | 41,399 |
| Apoprotein* | 39,049 |
| Oligosaccharides | 2,114 |
| Retinal | 284 |
| Amino acids (no.) | 348 |
| Helical content | ~66% |
| Oligosaccharides (carbohydrates) | Mannose and *N*-acetyl glucosamine[†] |
| Amino acid bound to retinal | LYS No. 296 |
| Amino acids bound to phosphate | SER (near C-terminus) |
| Amino acids bound to oligosaccharides | ASP (near N-terminus) |

*Less retinal and the oligosaccharides.

[†]See Chapter 3 for structures.

(Adapted from Schichi H. *Biochemistry of Vision*. New York: Academic Press, 1983;118.)

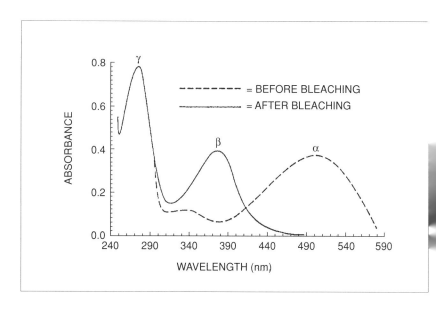

**FIGURE 1-18    The absorption spectrum of rhodopsin and opsin.**
The spectra of intermediate forms are not shown. The γ peak is characteristic of all proteins. (Adapted from C.D.B. Bridges. *Biochemistry of Vision. In* Graymore CN (ed.) *Biochemistry of the Eye.* New York: Academic Press, 1970; 571.

It has been known for many years that rhodopsin has certain spectral or light-absorbing properties. Figure 1-18 shows the absorption spectrum of frog rhodopsin before and after exposure to light; that is, before and after rhodopsin is converted to retinal and opsin. This process is also called the *bleaching* of rhodopsin. Three peaks are seen. The α-peak is the absorption of 11-*cis* retinal bound to opsin (as rhodopsin). The β-peak is the absorption of all-*trans* retinal that is not bound to opsin. The γ-peak (280 nm) is the *protein absorption peak* common to both opsin and rhodopsin. The shifting of these absorption signals led investigators to discover the intermediate forms of rhodopsin and its final products in the bleaching process. The conversion of rhodopsin to opsin, however, is only the tip of the iceberg of visual transduction. In Chapter 6 the remainder of the process is described.

Rhodopsin is the visual transduction protein of rod photoreceptors, whose role is principally visual sensation. Color vision, however, is realized by light transduction involving proteins in cone photoreceptors, of which there are three types: blue-, green-, and red-absorbing proteins. These photoreceptors are maximally sensitive, respectively, at wavelengths of 440 to

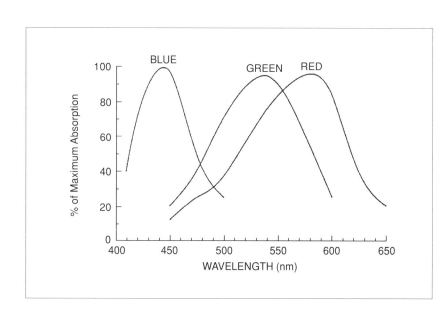

**FIGURE 1-19    Absorption maxima of the blue, green, and red pigment proteins of the cones of the retina.**
These proteins bind to 11-cis retinal in the same manner as opsin does. However, the amino acid sequences vary from opsin to absorb light at different wavelengths.

450 nm, 535 to 555 nm, and 570 to 590 nm (Figure 1-19). The proteins contained in these cones have not been characterized as well as rhodopsin, but the chromophore that acts as the prosthetic group in each is also 11-*cis* retinal. It is known that approximately 50% of the amino acid sequence of each cone protein is identical to that of rhodopsin (Nathans, 1987). Furthermore, the portion of the cone's transducing proteins that crosses the membrane also has α-helical forms. Color-blind persons usually lack one or two types of these cone proteins.

## Mucous Glycoproteins

Glycoproteins are proteins to which small chains of sugars (or carbohydrates) are bound. Rhodopsin is an example of one glycoprotein. Such proteins are to be distinguished from *proteoglycans*, in which the carbohydrates are the dominant structures (see Chapter 3). Glycoproteins have a variety of roles which include structure orientation, immune recognition, and biologic lubrication. In the precorneal tear film, the mucoid layer (and to a lesser extent, the aqueous layer), contains mucous glycoproteins, *mucins*. These proteins are similar to the mucins found in other mucous secreting tissues such as the gastrointestinal tract, nasal passages, and trachea.

Mucins typically contain larger amounts of carbohydrates than serum and plasma membrane glycoproteins. However, the carbohydrates and the way that they are attached to the proteins differ substantially from those carbohydrates found in proteoglycans. The carbohydrates are attached in numerous short chains along the length of the polypeptide chain unit (Figure 1-20, top). Each peptide chain unit containing carbohydrates is separated by a short length of peptide chain having no carbohydrates. This results in a heterogeneous molecule like that shown at the bottom of Figure 1-20. Berta and Török (1986) stated that typically there is a significant proportion of the amino acid proline in these proteins, and this seems to support the random nature of their structures. Representative molecular

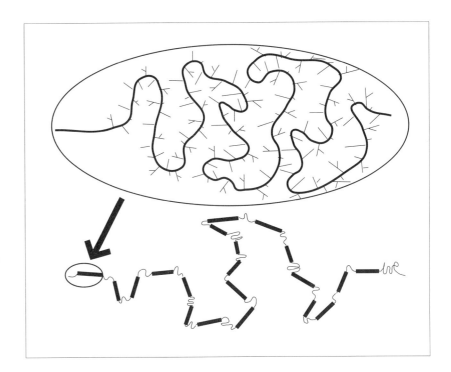

**FIGURE 1-20    Molelcular diagram of a mucin protein of the precorneal tear film.**
The top portion is an enlargement of a section of the molecule. In the enlargement, segments of the twisted polypeptide chain have short carbohydrate chains (oligosaccharides) bound to them (*thin lines*). Intervening segments have no oligosaccharides (shown below). (Adapted from Berta and Török, 1986)

weights of nonocular mucins are 0.5 to 16 × 10$^5$ d. About 55% of the composition of ocular mucins is carbohydrates. The composition and linkages of these carbohydrates are discussed in Chapter 3.

Ocular mucins are secreted principally by the conjunctival goblet cells. They maintain the stability of the tear film; act as a biologic lubricant at the epithelial surface; and are a viscoelastic buffer against mechanical shock. Mucins support tear film stability by trapping lipids within their structure. Several pathological conditions will cause mucins to become decreased or absent from the tear film, for example, vitamin A deficiency, ocular pemphigoid (conjunctival alterations), Stevens-Johnson syndrome (an acute, severe symptom complex that involves the mucous membranes and skin), and alkali burns. All these conditions destroy the goblet cells and interrupt mucin production, which results in rapid breakup of the tear film. This occurs even though there is an adequate volume of the aqueous layer of tears.

## Collagen

Collagen is a protein of great structural importance to the eye just as it is for other parts of the body. Approximately 80% to 90% of the bulk of the eye contains collagen. This protein is an extracellular, insoluble molecular complex that has a variety of morphologic roles. Collagens act as supporting members or fibers to form and maintain tissue structure (including wound repair), as scaffolding upon which basement membrane is constructed, as extracellular skeletons, and as devices to anchor cells onto acellular areas. In the eye collagen also makes up the semi-liquid gel of the vitreous humor.

**TABLE 1-6   Types of Collagen in Ocular Tissues**

| Type | Major Molecular Species (Chain Types) | Molecular Characteristics | Ocular Sites | Function |
|------|------|------|------|------|
| I | [α1(I)]$_2$, α2(I) | Low content of hydroxylysine, low content of carbohydrate | Corneal stroma, sclera | Structural fibers |
| II | [α1(II)]$_3$ | High content of hydroxylysine, high content of carbohydrate | Cornea, sclera, vitreous | Structural fibers |
| III | [α1(III)]$_3$ | High content of hydroxyproline, low content of hydroxylysine, low content of carbohydrate | Blood vessels, cornea, iris, lids | Limits diameter of fibers and repairs fibers |
| IV | [α1(IV)]$_2$, α2(IV) | High content of hydroxylysine, high content of carbohydrate, terminal ends retained | Descemet's membrane, lens capsule, capillaries | Amorphous or basement membrane scaffold |
| V | [α1(V)]$_2$, α2(V) | High content of hydroxylysine, high content of carbohydrate | Corneal stroma, endothelium | Limits diameter of fiber and cell shape |
| VI | [α1(VI), α2(VI), α3(VI)] | Two substantial noncollagen sequences at each end | Corneal stroma | Adhesion |
| VII | [α1(VII)]$_3$ | Forms antiparallel fibers | Anchoring fibrils of Bowman's membrane | Adhesion |
| VIII | [α1(VIII), α2(VIII), α3(VIII)] | Low content of hydroxylysine, low content of hydroxproline, noncollagenous sequences at each end | Descemet's membrane | Scaffold of basement membrane |

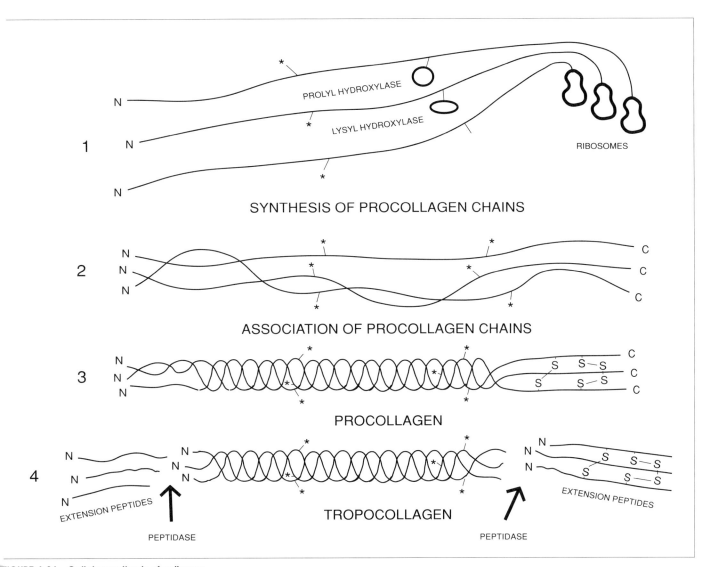

1

N

PROLYL HYDROXYLASE

N

LYSYL HYDROXYLASE

N

RIBOSOMES

SYNTHESIS OF PROCOLLAGEN CHAINS

2

N
N
N

C
C
C

ASSOCIATION OF PROCOLLAGEN CHAINS

3

N
N
N

S  S—S
S  S—S

C
C
C

PROCOLLAGEN

4

N
N
N

N
N
N

N
N

S  S—S
S  S—S

EXTENSION PEPTIDES

EXTENSION PEPTIDES

PEPTIDASE

TROPOCOLLAGEN

PEPTIDASE

**FIGURE 1-21  Cellular synthesis of collagen.**
(1) Single collagen chains are synthesized, as are all proteins, in the usual manner, on ribosomes. During synthesis some of the lysine and proline amino acids have hydroxyl groups added to them. (2) After synthesis three chains associate together along common hydrophobic areas. (3) The formation of disulfide bonds (at the C-terminal areas) causes the three chains to wrap around each other in a triple helix. Note that the ends of the molelcules do not form a helix. This procollagen form is ready for transport outside the cell. (4) Synthesis of the unit (known as tropocollagen) is complete with the hydrolysis of the N- and C- extension peptides. Non–fiber forming collagens, however, do not lose their extension peptides. (Adapted from McGilvery RW. *Biochemistry, A Functional Approach*. Philadelphia: W.B. Saunders, 1983;168.)

Miller and Gay (1990) have described 13 different types of collagen. At present, at least 12 types have been found in the eye. (Eight are shown in Table 1-6).

Collagen is a protein complex whose basic unit consists of a triple helix (*tropocollagen*) of three polypeptide chains wound around each other like the strands of a rope. These units make up part of a larger assembly (described later). The helical form of the unit chains is different from an α-helix. In fact, there exists both a helical structure for each chain (minor helix) and a helical structure formulated by the three chains together (major helix). The molecular weight of a single tropocollagen unit of type I collagen is 400 kd.

The assembled structures of collagen molecules are best understood in terms of how cells make them. Like all protein synthesis, collagen peptide synthesis occurs by "reading" of a specific code (sequence) from messenger RNA at ribosomes located along the cell's rough endoplasmic reticulum. Collagens also undergo posttranslational modifications during and after synthesis (Figure 1-21). In Step 1 of the figure, each of the three chains being assembled contains substantial amounts of the amino acids proline and lysine, as indicated by small lines protruding from each chain. These amino acids are partly hydroxylated during peptide synthesis by the catalytic action of hydroxylase enzymes. The added hydroxyl groups are indicated by asterisks in the figure. In addition, the major portion of each chain contains glycine as every third amino acid. As it is, the frequent occurrence of the small glycine molecule is necessary to fit the three chains within a triple helical structure. The next events occur at Steps 2 and 3, in which the three chains become associated hydrophobically. They also form disulfide bonds at their C-terminal regions and then with a zipperlike motion, rapidly twist into a triple helix, with the hydroxyl groups protruding outward. The triple helix is stabilized by interchain hydrogen bonding in which the hydroxyl groups also participate. Some of the hydroxyl groups subsequently become bound to small sugar chains (oligosaccharides), though the reason for this is unknown. In the fiber-forming collagens (types I, II, III, and V), and similarly in some other types, large portions of the nonhelical N- and C-terminal peptides (*extension peptides*) are removed by the catalytic action of peptidase enzymes.

The remaining structure, shown in Step 4, is *tropocollagen*. Tropocollagen formation takes place after the secretion of procollagen to the outside surface of the cell. Some evidence indicates that the extension peptides regulate the synthesis of new procollagen chains (Miller and Gay, 1990). The scaffold-associated type IV collagen is not subject to the molecular truncation of Step 4. The kinds of polypeptides (i.e., the sequences) that compose tropocollagen may be similar (*homopolymeric*) or dissimilar (*heteropolymeric*). Type I collagen is heteropolymeric and consists of two α1(I) chains and one α2(I) chain, designated [α1(I)]$_2$ α2(I), whereas type II collagen is homopolymeric and consists of three α1(III) chains designated: [α1(III)]$_3$ (see Table 1-6).

Once outside the cell, the tropocollagen units go through a process of assembly near the cell surface. The process consists in the lateral association of tropocollagen units, which are staggered lengthwise in three-dimensional space (Figure 1-22). This association is made up of hydrophobic interactions and the formed cross-links of lysine and hydroxylysine, as shown by the slanted vertical lines of the microfibril. Cross-linking adds considerable strength to the growing fibers. The microfibril is an association of five staggered lengths of collagen units. The next larger unit, the collagen fibril, is made up of many microfibrils whose diameters range from 10 to

**FIGURE 1-22   Collagen fiber formation.**
Tropocollagen units associate hydrophobically and are strengthened by covalent cross-links (*small lines in the microfibril*). Note that the units are staggered with open spaces between the ends of the units. Electron micrographs of these fibrils and fibers show a banded pattern (as indicated for the fibril) in which the electron-dense material enters the spaces, making them appear dark. A microfibril consists of five rows of cross-linked tropocollagens. A fibril is arbitrarily defined as being 10 to 300 nm in diameter. A fiber is composed of several fibrils.

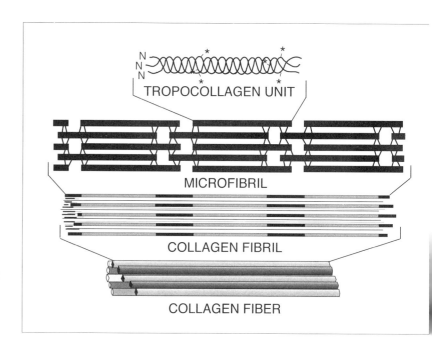

TROPOCOLLAGEN UNIT

MICROFIBRIL

COLLAGEN FIBRIL

COLLAGEN FIBER

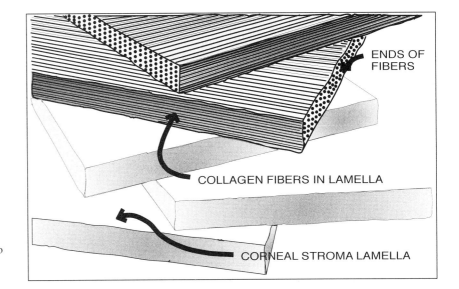

FIGURE 1-23    Collagen fibers in the lamellae of the corneal stroma (predominately type I collagen).

The long axes of fibers in adjacent lamellae are run at angles to one another. (Adapted from Hogan MJ, Alvarado JA, and Weddell JE. *Histology of the Human Eye.* Philadelphia: W.B. Saunders, 1971;92.)

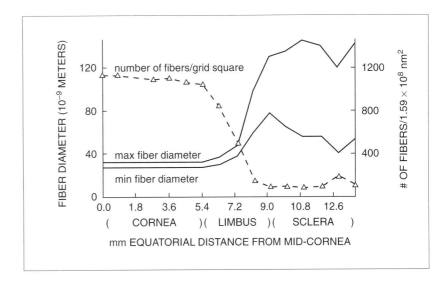

FIGURE 1-24    Fiber diameter as a function of distance from the central cornea.

It can be seen that stromal fibers are small, regular, and numerous in comparison to those in the sclera. This contributes to the clarity of the cornea. Proteoglycans and collagen fiber organization in human corneoscleral tissue. (Adapted from Borcherding MS et al. *Exp Eye Res* 1975;21:59–71.)

300 nm, depending on collagen type and tissue location. The association of several fibrils is termed a *fiber.*

## Ocular, Structural Roles

Fiber structures take on many forms. In the corneal stroma the fibers form sheets (*lamellae*) whose long axes are parallel within the sheet, but in adjacent lamellae lie at different angles (Figure 1-23). Such a structure confers considerable cross-sectional strength on the cornea. This stromal collagen is described by Borcherding et al. (1975) as having fibers with a uniform diameter of about 30 nm. In comparison, adjacent scleral collagen fiber diameters vary between 40 and 140 nm (Figure 1-24). The majority of this collagen is type I (see Table 1-6). However, type III collagen has also been reported to be present with sufficient enough frequency (Cintron et al., 1988) that it must have some importance. Two roles have been suggested for type III. Some think it participates in establishing fibers during wound healing. More recently others believe it may control the diameter of the fibers. This is especially important for maintaining corneal clarity. It might accomplish this by assuming an exterior conformation that prevents attachment of additional fibrils (Miller and Gay, 1990).

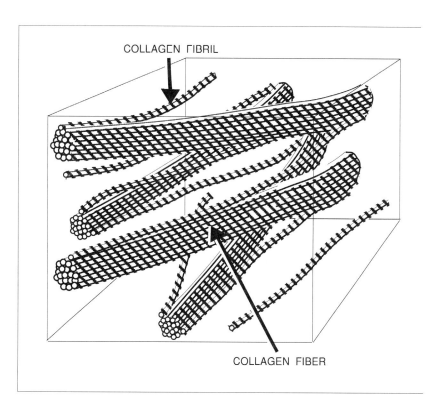

COLLAGEN FIBRIL

COLLAGEN FIBER

**FIGURE 1-25   Three-dimensional representation of a cross section of the vitreous gel.**
The gel is predominately composed of (1) type II collagen *fibers* of low density and (2) hyaluronic acid (not shown). A limited number of collagen *fibrils* also occurs. Ninety-nine percent of the gel is water. (Adpated from Sebag J, and Balazs EA. Morphology and ultrastructure of human vitreous fibers. *Invest Ophthalmol Vis Sci* 1989;30:1867–1871.

An entirely different collagen structure occurs in the ocular vitreous (Figure 1-25). In the gellike milieu of the vitreous, collagen fibers are arranged in parallel, extending across the entire volume of secondary vitreous from the anterior to the posterior aspect (Sebag and Balazs, 1989). At a few locations somewhat random fibrils are seen joining the fibers. The fibers establish firm attachments of the vitreous to its surrounding tissues (most notably in the vicinity of the ora serrata and the macula). Vitreal collagen, classified as type II (Snowden and Swann, 1980), is also known as *vitrosin.* Some differences in vitreal type II collagen suggest that it may retain portions of its extension peptides. More recently, type IX collagen was found on the surface of type II collagen in vitreous (Brewton et al., 1991). This collagen is thought to control the diameter of type II fibers. The space between collagen fibers and vitreal fibrils is occupied by large polymeric sugars known as *proteoglycans* (Chapter 3).

The collagen found in basement membrane structures (Descemet's, Bowman's, lens capsule, ocular blood vessels), is predominantly type IV, except in Descemet's, where it is type VIII (Kapoor et al., 1986). Its structure is flexible in comparison with those collagens found in fibers. An analogy to a box-spring mattress is appropriate. It should be reemphasized that type IV collagen does not lose any extension peptides during posttranslational modification. These nonhelical regions are capable of forming bonds with other type IV collagens in geometric arrays. This is also true of type VIII collagen, where it occurs. Accordingly, Miller and Gay (1990) have described the important end-to-end bonds that result in an open, meshlike network. Though the structure is difficult to visualize Figure 1-26 indicates two possible geometric forms for types IV and VIII collagens. The hexagonal form was described by Miller and Gay. The tetragon approximates a basic form for the suggested structure of Descemet's membrane (see Figure 1-26) that resembles that seen on electron micrographs obtained by Jakus (1964).

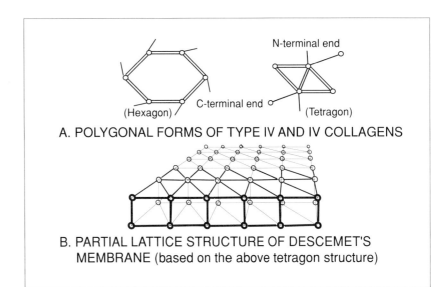

A. POLYGONAL FORMS OF TYPE IV AND IV COLLAGENS

B. PARTIAL LATTICE STRUCTURE OF DESCEMET'S
MEMBRANE (based on the above tetragon structure)

**FIGURE 1-26** (*A*) Type VIII collagen and (*B*) Descemet's membrane.

Descemet's membrane is a basement membrane with a lattice structure whose units are similar to the tetragon shape in the upper right-hand corner of the figure.

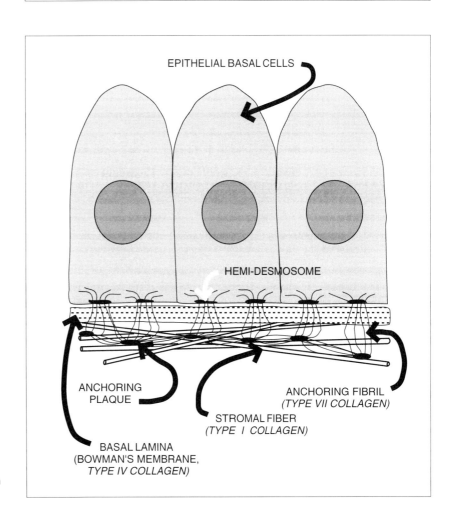

**FIGURE 1-27** Anchoring fibrils (type VII collagen) attach epithelial basal cells to the outermost stromal lamella.

A fourth structural type found in ocular tissue is the anchoring fibril. Anchoring fibrils can be observed extending between the basal epithelial cells of the cornea and the outermost lamellae of the corneal stroma. The fibers extend through Bowman's membrane and serve to attach the epithelium to the stroma (Figure 1-27). Type VII collagen has been identified (Gipson et al., 1987) with these fibrils. The type I collagen fibers in the most anterior lamellae (see Figure 1-27) are oriented somewhat randomly. The anchoring fibers are attached from the hemidesmosomes of the epithelia basal cells to anchoring plaques on the stromal fibers. Other anchoring fibrils extend from one anchoring plaque to the next. It is thought that in diabetes the synthesis of altered anchoring fibrils results in loose adhesion of the epithelium to its underlying stroma (Kenyon, 1979).

## Summary

Proteins in ocular tissue have a wide variety of functional roles. Though the number of proteins in the eye is huge, some deserve special attention. Crystallins are soluble lens proteins whose normal function is supportive in the maintenance of elongated lens fiber cells. These proteins are thought to be involved in the manifestation of senile cortical cataracts by the oxidation of the disulfide bonds, though the process is incompletely understood. Cross-linked proteins (not disulfide bonded) have also been implicated in the formation of nuclear cataracts. Rhodopsin and cone pigment proteins act as the initial participants in phototransduction. They are membrane proteins found on the discs of rods and cones. Vitamin A aldehyde (retinal) is a prosthetic group on these proteins whose release triggers the cascade of phototransduction. Mucous glycoproteins known as mucins are found in the precorneal tear film (mucous layer) and act to stabilize the tear film. Collagen, the principal type of ocular protein, is found in 80% to 90% of the bulk of the eye. From basic tropocollagen units it forms complex structure that may form fibers, ground substance, or anchoring rods. It is also a constituent of the gel of the vitreous humor.

## References

Berbers GAM, Boerman OC, Bloemandal H, and de Jong WM. Primary gene products of bovine beta-crystallin and association behavior of its aggregates. *Eur J Biochem* 1982;25:495–502.

Berta A, and Török M. Soluble glycoproteins in aqueous tears. *In* Holly FJ (ed). *The Preocular Tear Film.* Lubbock, Texas: Dry Eye Institute, 1986; 506–521.

Borcherding MS, Blacik LJ, Sittig RA, Bizzelli JW, Breen M, and Weinstein HG. Proteoglycans and collagen fibre organization in human corneoscleral tissue. *Exp Eye Res* 1975;21:59–70.

Bours J, and Hockwin O. Artunterschiede bei Linsenproteinen nach Trennung mit Isolekktrofukussiering auf Polyacrylamid-Dünnschich platten. *Berl Munch Tieraerztl Wochenshr* 1976;89:417–422.

Brewton RG, Wright DW, and Mayne R. Structural and functional comparison of type IX collagen-proteoglycan from chicken cartilage and vitreous humor. *J Biol Chem* 1991;266:4752–4757.

Bridges CDB. Biochemistry of vision. *In* Graymore CN (ed). *Biochemistry of the Eye.* New York: Academic Press, 1970;563–644.

Chao C-CW, Butala SM, and Herp A. Studies on the isolation and composition of human ocular mucin. *Exp Eye Res* 1988;47:185–196.

Chiesa R, McDermott MJ, and Spector A. Differential synthesis and phosphorylation of the alpha-crystallin A and B chains during bovine lens fiber cell differentiation. *Curr Eye Res* 1989;8:151–158.

Cintron C, Hong B-S, Covington HI, and Macarak EJ. Heterogeneity of collagens in rabbit cornea: Type III collagen. *Invest Ophthalmol Vis Sci* 1988;29:767–775.

Dilley KJ, and Pirie A. Changes to the proteins of the human lens nucleus in cataract. *Exp Eye Res* 1974;19:59–72.

Dillon J, Spector A, and Nakanishi K. Identification of beta-carbolines isolated from fluorescent human lens proteins. *Nature* 1976;259:422–423.

Farnsworth P, Kamosinski T, King G, and Groth-Vaselli. Predicted 3-D structure of alpha-crystallin subunits using molecular dynamics provides a working model. *Invest Ophthalmol Vis Sci* 1993;34:1412.

Garcia-Castineiras S, Dillon J, and Spector A. Non-tryptophan fluorescence associated with human lens protein; apparent complexity and isolation of bityrosine and anthranilic acid. *Exp Eye Res* 1978;26:461–476.

Garner MH, and Spector A. Selective oxidation of cysteine and methionine in normal and senile cataractous lenses. *Proc Natl Acad Sci USA* 1980; 77:1274–1277.

Gipson IK, Spurr-Mauchaud SJ, and Tisdale AS. Anchoring fibrils form a complex network in human and rabbit cornea. *Invest Ophthalmol Vis Sci* 1987;28:212–220.

Harding JJ. Changes in lens proteins in cataract. *In* Bloemendal H (ed). *Molecular and Cellular Biology of the Eye.* New York: John Wiley & Sons, 1981;327–365.

Harding JJ, and Crabbe MJC. The lens: Development, proteins, metabolism and cataract. *In* Davson H (ed). *The Eye*, 3rd ed. Orlando: Academic Press, 1984;207–492.

Hoenders HJ, and Bloemendal H. Aging of lens proteins. *In* Bloemendal H (ed). *Molecular and Cellular Biology of the Eye Lens.* New York: John Wiley & Sons, 1981;279–326.

Horwitz J. The function of alpha-crystallin. *Invest Ophthalmol Vis Sci* 1993;34:10–22.

Jakus, M. *Ocular Fine Structure. Selected Electron Micrographs.* Boston: Little, Brown, 1964.

Jose, JG. The lens. *In* Anderson RE (ed). *Biochemistry of the Eye.* San Francisco: American Academy of Ophthalmology, 1983;111–144.

Kapoor R, Bornstein P, and Sage H. Type VIII collagen from bovine Descemet's membrane: Structural characterization of a triple-helical domain. *Biochemistry* 1986;25:3930–3937.

Kenyon KR. Recurrent corneal erosion: Pathogenesis and therapy. *Int Ophthalmol Clin* 1979;19:169.

Lerman S, and Borkman R. Spectroscopic evaluation and classification of the normal, aging, and cataractous lens. *Ophthalmic Res* 1976;8:335–353.

Miller E., and Gay S. *In* Cohen K, Dieglemann R, and Lindbard W (eds). *Wound Healing.* Philadelphia: WB Saunders, 1990;130–151.

Nathans J. Molecular biology of visual pigments. *Ann Rev Neurosci* 1987;10:163–194.

Pirie A. Formation of $N'$-formylkynurenine in proteins from lens and other sources by exposure to sunlight. *Biochem J* 1971;125:203–208.

Pirie A. Fluorescence of $N'$-formylkynurenine and of proteins exposed to sunlight. *Biochem J* 1972;128;1365–1367.

Sebag J, and Balazs EA. Morphology and ultrastructure of human vitreous fibers. *Invest Ophthalmol Vis Sci* 1989; 30: 1867–1871.

Snowden JM, and Swann DA. Vitreous structure. V. The morphology and thermal stability of vitreous collagen fibers and comparison to articular cartilage (type II) collagen. *Invest Ophthalmol Vis Sci* 1980;19:610–618.

Spector A. The search for a solution to senile cataracts. *Invest Ophthalmol Vis Sci* 1984;25:130–146.

Stryer L. *Biochemistry*, 3rd ed. Orlando: Academic Press, 1988.

Summers LJ, Blundell TL, Gause GG, and Tomarov SI. A computer graphics model of frog γ-crystallin based on the three-dimensional structure of calf γ·II crystallin. *FEBS Letters* 1986;208:11–16.

Truscott RJW, Faull K, and Augusteyn RC. The identification of anthranilic acid in proteolytic digests of cataractous lens proteins. *Ophthalmic Res* 1977;9:263–268.

van Heyningen LR. Experimental studies on cataract. *Invest Ophthalmol* 1976;15:685–697.

Wald G. The molecular basis of visual excitation. *Nature* 1968;219:800–807.

Weiter JJ, and Finch ED. Ultraviolet light and human cataract. *Nature* 1975;257:71–72.

Wistow GJ, and Piatigorsky J. Lens crystallins: The evaluation and expression of proteins for a highly specialized tissue. *Ann Rev Biochem* 1988:57:479–504.

# Chapter 2

# Enzymes

## Review of Enzymology

Enzymes are proteins that possess the ability to optimize the rates of biochemical reactions in cellular tissues. Since they remain unaltered, they are true chemical catalysts. Their intervention in cellular metabolic reactions is essential to the survival and operation of every class of cells in the body. Accordingly, enzymes are involved in thousands of cellular reactions, from the conversion of glucose into cellular energy to the very formation of enzymes themselves. In the eye, enzymes are also instrumental in the visual transduction process, the generation of intraocular pressure, the maintenance of a clear cornea (deturgescence), the destruction of bacteria in the precorneal tear film, the development of lens fiber cells, and many other functions that support vision. At normal cellular temperatures (37°C), and especially in the somewhat cooler regions of the cornea (30° to 35°C), biochemical reactions would virtually cease without enzymes.

Kinetically, an enzyme (or any catalyst) increases the rate of a reaction by lowering the amount of energy required (i.e., the activation energy) to convert a reactant (substrate) into a product (Figure 2-1). In the case of an enzyme, at least one intermediate is formed prior to product formation. The advantage of an enzyme-catalyzed reaction is the comparatively small amounts of energy required ($Y_1 + Y_2$) to form the product versus that needed ($X$) when no catalyst is present. Therefore, $(Y_1 + Y_2) << X$. These reactions are usually reversible, which means that a large amount of substrate (A) will drive the reaction to form product (C), and vice versa.

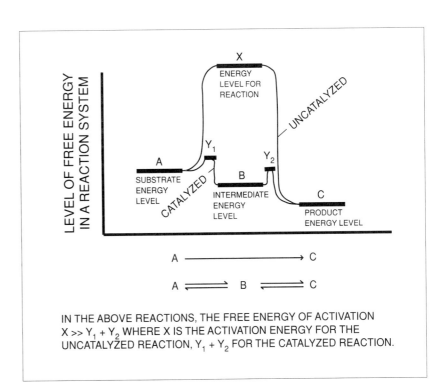

**FIGURE 2-1  Free energy levels in enzymatic and nonenzymatic reactions.**
Enzyme-catalyzed reactions have two small energy-driven steps between the formation of an intermediate (B) and a product (C).

In a series of enzyme driven reactions, usually one reaction tends to proceed in a given direction and the enzyme involved is called the *rate-limiting enzyme*. On the molecular level, what actually occurs in an enzyme-catalyzed reaction is that the substrate (Figure 2-2) becomes bound to a region of the enzyme known as the *active site*. This is usually a cleft or a small cave in the structure of the catalytic protein. The molecular architecture of this site is suitable for holding the substrate in an orientation favorable for conversion, first to an intermediate and then to a product. Small changes to the enzyme (e.g., transfer of protons, conformational strain) occur as part of the catalytic event, but the enzyme is always returned to its original form at the end of each reaction (i.e., it is unchanged).

Enzymes, like proteins, may be classified by several criteria. One criterion is based on the kinds of reactions supported: oxidoreduction, transfer of molecular groups, hydrolytic cleavage, double-bond alteration, isomerization, or condensation (ligation). On a kinetic basis, the classifications of Michaelis-Menten and allosteric types give a better idea of what enzymes actually do.

## Michaelis-Menten Enzymes

Michaelis-Menten enzymes have functional properties that were described mathematically by Henri in 1903, by Leonor Michaelis and Maude Menten in 1913, and, finally in 1925, by G. E. Briggs and J. B. S. Haldane (Palmer, 1981). The reaction kinetics are derived from the equation

$$[E] + [S] \underset{k_2}{\overset{k_1}{\rightleftharpoons}} [ES] \overset{k_3}{\rightarrow} [P] \tag{2-1}$$

in which $[E]$, $[S]$, $[ES]$ and $[P]$ are the molar concentrations of enzyme, substrate, enzyme-substrate complex, and product, respectively, and $k_1$, $k_2$, and $k_3$ are the rates for each conversion to and from $[ES]$. When in brackets the terms refer specifically to their molar concentrations. The concentration relationships for these conversions over time may be visualized in Figure 2-3. Notice that the enzyme becomes saturated very early with substrate

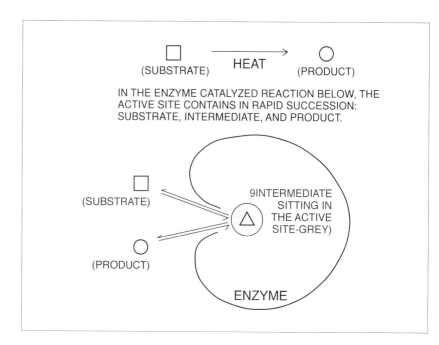

**FIGURE 2-2   Basic diagram of an enzymatic catalyzed reaction compared to a nonenzymatic catalyzed reaction.**
Noncatalyzed reactions are often driven by heat, whereas enzyme-catalyzed reactions align and hold reactants (substrates) at the active site for reactions to occur.

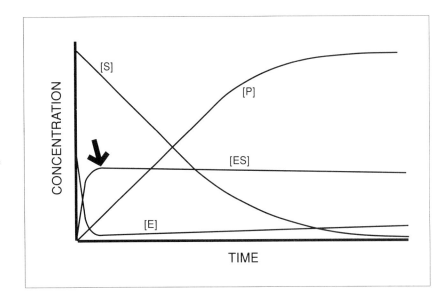

FIGURE 2-3 Concentration levels of the components of an enzymatic catalyzed reaction versus time.
The concentration of the enzyme-substrate complex ([ES], *arrow*) is held nearly constant as the substrate ([S]) is consumed and the product ([P]) is formed. This is another way of saying that the enzyme's active site is saturated. Note that the decrease in free enzyme concentration [E] is indirectly proportional to the increase in [ES]. Adapted from Mathews CK, and van Holde KE. *Biochemistry.* Redwood City, Calif.: Benjamin/Cummings. 1990;359.

(enzyme-substrate complex [ES]) and remains at a fairly steady level. Accordingly, the change in [ES] with time may be described as

$$\frac{d\,[ES]}{dt} \cong 0. \tag{2-2}$$

Since the change in [ES] is very small or nearly zero, $d[ES]/dt$ may also be described in terms that cause its formation, $k_1\,[E][S]$, and its dissolution, $-(k_2\,[ES] + k_3[ES])$. Moreover, these terms may also be made nearly equal to zero, rearranged, and substituted in the following first-order reaction equation:

$$\text{Velocity} = v = k_3[ES] \tag{2-3}$$

to yield the equation

$$v = \frac{V_{max}[S]}{[S] + K_m} \tag{2-4}$$

where $V_{max}$ is the maximum velocity of the enzyme

and $K_m = \dfrac{k_2 + k_3}{k_1}$ = Michaelis-Menten constant

The derivation of Equation 2–4 is given in the Glossary under *velocity*. Equations 2–3 and 2–4 are both rate equations. The latter, known as the *Michaelis-Menten equation*, defines the maximum velocity ($V_{max}$) and the dissociation constant ($K_m$) of an enzyme. These terms are useful for measuring the rate properties of an enzyme and comparing the relative affinity ("stickiness") of different substrates for the same enzyme. The Michaelis constant is, however, actually a *dissociation constant* for the [ES] complex: $[ES] \rightarrow [E] + [S]$. Since this term is opposite in meaning to *affinity*, one must be aware that the lower the $K_m$ value, the greater will be the affinity of substrate and enzyme, provided that $k_3$ is sufficiently small. Sometimes this is not the case, and enzymologists have used the term "apparent $K_m$" to indicate this. (For more details on the meaning of $K_m$ readers can consult the discussion by Mathews and van Holde [1990]).

The $K_m$ is also equal to the substrate concentration $[S]$ when $v$ is $1/2\ V_{max}$ (Figure 2-4). For most enzymes, $K_m$ lies between the substrate concentrations of $1 \times 10^{-1}$ and $1 \times 10^{-7}\,M$ (Stryer, 1988). Generally, the $V_{max}$ and the $K_m$ of an enzyme are not measured by constructing graphs like that in Figure 2-4, because of the difficulty in obtaining the value of $V_{max}$ as it approaches an asymptotic limit.

Another approach to finding $V_{max}$ and $K_m$ is to use a double-reciprocal plot such as a Lineweaver-Burk plot (Figure 2-5). The plot is constructed by using the reciprocal of the Michaelis-Menten equation:

$$\frac{1}{v} = \frac{1}{V_{max}} + \frac{K_m}{V_{max}} \cdot \frac{1}{[S]} \tag{2-5}$$

in order to obtain a straight line graph having two intercepts ($x$ and $y$), which give the reciprocal values for $K_m$ and $V_{max}$. In the eye, aldose reductase, which is involved in the formation of sugar cataracts, serves as an example of a Michaelis-Menten enzyme.

## Allosteric Enzymes

The word "allosteric" means *other site* and refers to the fact that the kinetics of these enzymes is influenced by substances bound to the enzyme at locations other than the active site or a single active site. This can occur in two different ways. Since allosteric enzymes are proteins with quaternary structures (i.e., they consist of more than one polypeptide chain), each chain has its own active site. When only one or a few active sites are occupied, the affinity of enzyme and substrate is low. In this situation, the velocity of the reaction is also slow. As the number of active sites occupied increases, the velocity increases, due to a conformational change in the protein that becomes more favorable to substrate affinity. The change is described as proceeding from a T (T = tense) form to an R (R = relaxed) form.

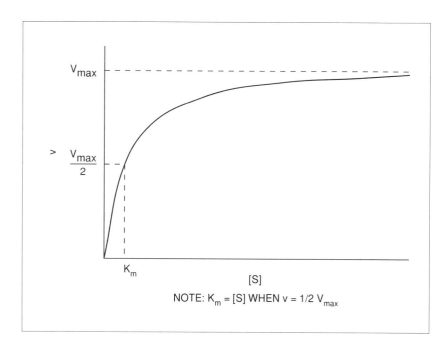

**FIGURE 2-4    A plot of enzyme velocity (V) versus substrate concentration [S].**
The velocity of the enzyme increases with [S] but never quite reaches its $V_{max}$. At one-half of $V_{max}$, one can measure the affinity of the enzyme for the substrate $K_m$.

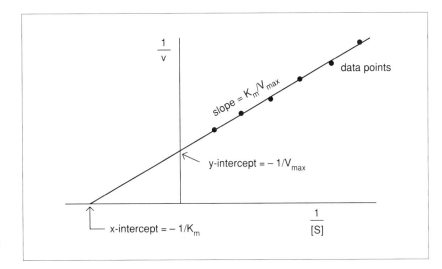

**FIGURE 2-5** A Lineweaver-Burk plot of $1/v$ (reciprocal of enzyme velocity) versus $1/[S]$ (reciprocal of the molar concentration of the substrate).
Enzyme velocities are measured in the concentration of substrate consumed or the product formed per unit time at stated conditions of temperature and bathing solutions. The term "units (U) of velocity" may also be used. Note that the $x$-intercept is a negative value.

A second way that the kinetics are influenced is with the binding of activator substances that occupy sites on the enzyme away from any of the active sites. In this way, such an enzyme is induced to change from its T form to its R form at much lower substrate concentrations. This is a biological way of "jump-starting" an enzyme to high velocities at lower substrate concentrations. Figure 2-6 shows a hypothetical enzyme in the two forms when occupied by activators or multiple substrates (inhibitors, also shown, are discussed later). Figure 2-7 indicates a graph of velocity versus [S] concentration for an allosteric enzyme without (on the right) and with (on the left) bound activator substances. Note that with such enzymes $K_m$ becomes known as $K_{apparent}$ (also referred to as $K_{app}$ or $K_{0.5}$), since the $K$ value is dependent on activators as well. In the eye sodium-potassium–activated adenosine triphosphatase (Na, K-ATPase), whose role is of special significance in the cornea and the ciliary body, serves as an example of an allosteric enzyme. When a Lineweaver-Burk plot is made of such enzymes (rather than Michaelis-Menten enzymes) it is nonlinear, and it may be difficult to determine $K_{app}$ (Figure 2-8). Other graphing techniques can be more useful, such as Eadie-Hofstee plots (Whikehart et al., 1987). These, however, are beyond the scope of this text.

## Enzyme Inhibition

Besides controlling the rates of enzymes positively (i.e., by stimulation), negative control may be imposed by inhibiting activity—either naturally, with substances within tissues, or artificially, with substances introduced into tissues. The latter represents a pharmacological technique that is useful, for example, in the treatment of glaucoma by inhibiting acetylcholinesterase, an enzyme that normally lyses acetylcholine in the autonomic nervous system.

Michaelis-Menten enzymes are usually inhibited by one of three mechanisms: *competitive*, *noncompetitive*, and *uncompetitive*. The pattern of Lineweaver-Burk plots in Figure 2-9 indicates how the apparent $K_m$ and $V_{max}$ may be influenced by the mechanism of inhibition. The expression $(1 + [I]/K_i)$ becomes a factor in all three forms of inhibition and may be used to determine the concentration of the inhibitor and its affinity for the enzyme. [I] represents the molar concentration of inhibitor, and $K_i$ is a measure of the

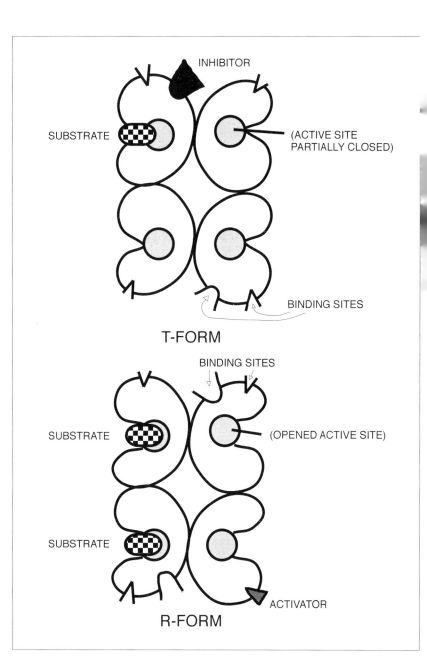

**FIGURE 2-6 Diagram of an allosteric enzyme in its T- and R forms.**

The enzyme is represented as four polypeptides with an active site (*gray circle*) in each polypeptide. In the T form the substrate has difficulty entering the active site, whereas in the R form access to the active site is easily gained. Inhibitors maintain these enzymes in their T forms, but activators convert them to their R forms. Substrates force a conformational change in the enzyme from T form to R form after enough substrates have entered the available active sites.

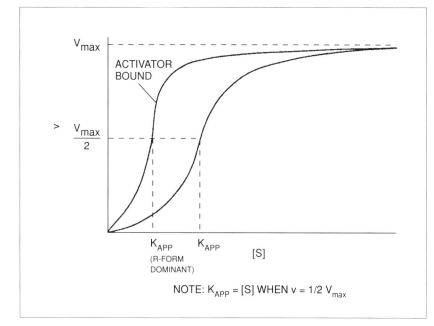

**FIGURE 2-7 The effect of an activator on the velocity and substrate affinity of an allosteric enzyme.**

When the activator is bound (left-hand curve), the apparent K is decreased (i.e., the affinity is increased) while the velocity is increased. This may be realized by drawing a vertical line through the two curves at a single concentration of [S].

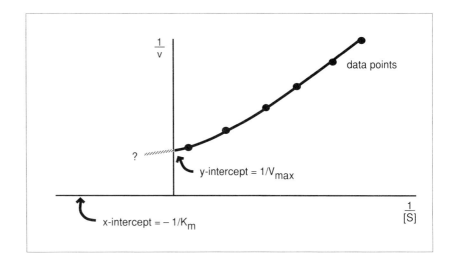

**FIGURE 2-8    Lineweaver-Burk plot of an allosteric enzyme.**
A Lineweaver-Burk plot does not yield accurate information about the apparent K of an allosteric enzyme. The degree of curvature is unknown.

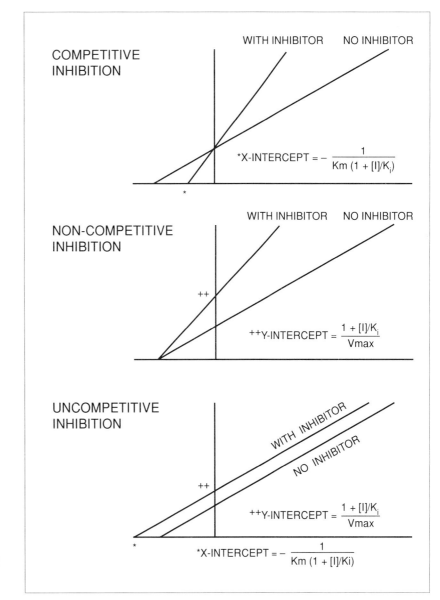

**FIGURE 2-9    Lineweaver-Burk plots for three inhibition mechanisms found in Michaelis-Menten enzymes.**
In competitive inhibition the apparent K is affected by competition of the inhibitor for the active site. In noncompetitive inhibition the velocity of the enzyme is affected by the proximity of the bound inhibitor to the active site. In uncompetitive inhibition both the apparent K (for one of the substrates) and the velocity of the enzyme are affected by the binding position of the inhibitor.

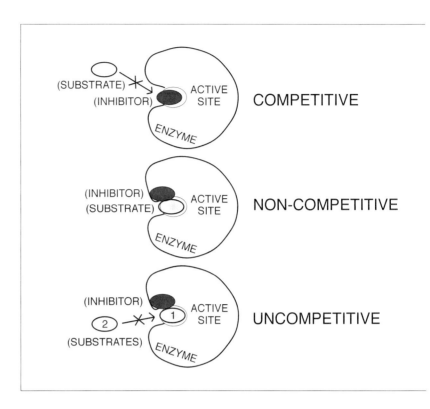

**FIGURE 2-10**  The binding positions and effects on enzyme catalysis produced by the three kinds of inhibition of Michaelis-Menten enzymes.
In competitive inhibition the substrate is blocked from entering the active site. In noncompetitive inhibition the substrate cannot easily be converted to product. In uncompetitive inhibition a second substrate is blocked from entering the active site.

affinity of the inhibitor for the enzyme in the same reciprocal sense as $K_m$ is for $[S]$. In *competitive inhibition,* the inhibitor replaces or competes with substrate for the active site. In *noncompetitive inhibition,* the inhibitor binds to a site close to the active site and prevents catalytic action on the substrate, even though it may bind to the enzyme. In *uncompetitive inhibition,* two substrates are usually required for catalytic action, and the inhibitor binds to an area close to the active site after the first substrate binds there. The inhibitor prevents the second substrate from binding. The latter mechanism occurs in the enzyme aldose reductase, which is involved in cataract formation in persons who have diabetes or galactosemia (Figure 2-10).

Allosteric enzymes are inhibited by substances binding to allosteric sites, which cause a conformational shift of the enzyme from its R form to its T form. In the T form it is more difficult for the substrate to bind to the enzyme (see Figures 2-6 and 2-11). Inhibition serves to slow down the rates of metabolic reactions. In a series of such reactions, the end product of the series may actually act as an inhibitor for the first reaction in that series (feedback inhibition). The hydrogen ion concentration (pH of the cellular environment) also influences enzyme reaction rates, both positively and negatively. Intracellular pH varies from one cell type to another and is not necessarily equivalent to the extracellular or "physiological" pH of 7.4. Most enzymes function intracellularly to control normal cell operation. Some act at cell membranes to facilitate transport, and a number also catalyze reactions extracellularly. Tear film lysozyme is an example of an extracellular enzyme.

## Lysozyme

Lysozyme is an enzyme of the precorneal tear film that is instrumental in destroying certain kinds of bacteria, namely, those that are positively stained with a crystal violet–iodine complex for peptidoglycans known as

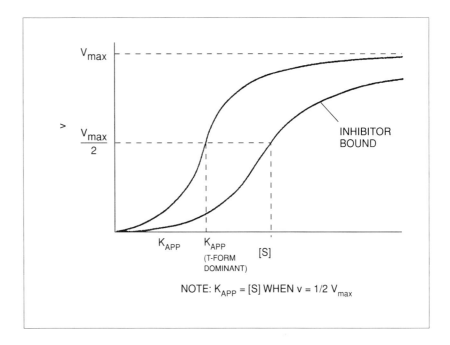

**◄FIGURE 2-11    Diagram of v vs. [S] when an inhibitor binds to an allosteric enzyme.**
The curve is shifted to the right causing both a decrease in velocity and a higher apparent K. The enzyme is in its T form, in the presence of an inhibitor.

NOTE: $K_{APP}$ = [S] WHEN v = 1/2 $V_{max}$

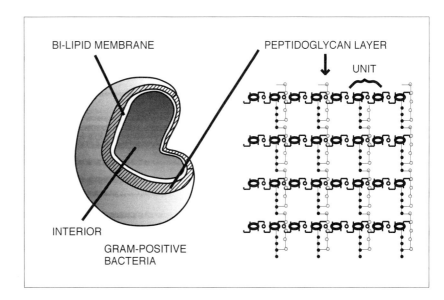

**FIGURE 2-12    Cutaway diagram of a Gram-positive bacterium, which has two boundary layers, a bilipid membrane, and a peptidoglycan layer.**
The latter, composed of a molecular cross-weaving of sugars and peptides, is represented on the right. A unit of two of the sugars is represented in Figure 2-13. (Adapted from Mathews CK, and van Holde KE. *Biochemistry.* Redwood City, Calif.: Benjamin/Cummings, 1990; 290.)

*Gram stain.* These "gram-positive bacteria" possess an outer coat of a peptide-glycan polymer (or peptidoglycan), which, in gram-negative bacteria, is only transiently stained since it is covered up by a second, outer lipid membrane. Lysozyme is able to hydrolyze or break up the glycan (sugar polymer) components of the peptidoglycan of gram-positive bacteria (Figure 2-12). The enzyme was initially described in 1922 by Alexander Fleming, a British bacteriologist (Stryer, 1988), who found it first in nasal mucous and later discovered that tears are a rich source of the enzyme. The concentration has been estimated to be 1.3 mg/mL of unstimulated tears (Sen and Sarin, 1980).

Specifically, the enzyme breaks the β1→4 glycosidic bond or oxygen bridge between the repeating glycan units of N-acetylmuramic acid (NAM) and N-acetylglucosamine (NAG) (Figure 2-13). Lysozyme is itself a globular protein with a molecular weight of about 14 kd. A portion of the bacterial peptidoglycan is able to fit in a groove on the outer face of the enzyme that contains the active site (Figure 2-14). This is an enzyme in which the

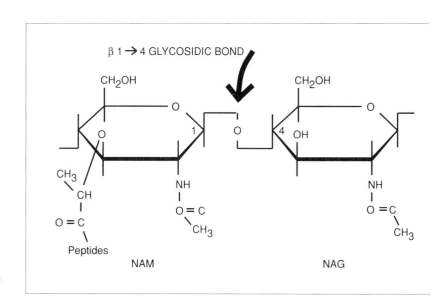

**FIGURE 2-13   The glycosidic bond of NAM and NAG units of a bacterial peptidoglycan.**

The basic two-sugar (carbohydrate) unit of bacterial peptidoglycans is composed of *N*-acetylmuramic acid (NAM) and *N*-acetylglucosamine (NAG). The two carbohydrates (and the ones that join them) are held together by an oxygen bridge (*arrow*) designated as a β1→4 glycosidic bond.

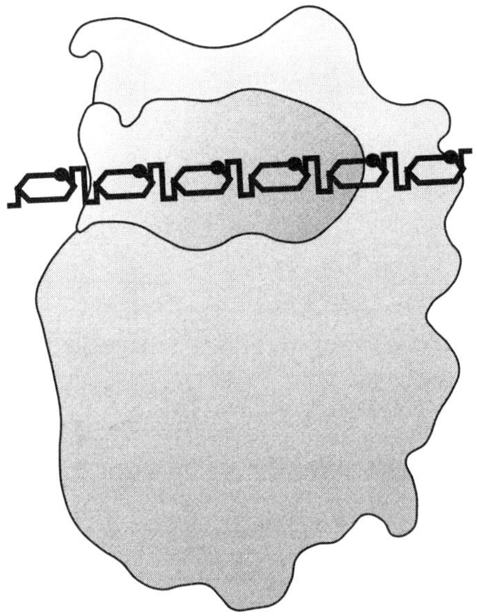

**FIGURE 2-14   Outline diagram of a lysozyme molecule.**

The enzyme has a groove (darker area near the top of the enzyme) into which the carbohydrate units of the peptidoglycans of bacteria can fit. Hydrolysis (or rupture) of the units occurs there. (Adapted from Lehninger AL. *Principles of Biochemistry.* New York: Worth, 1982; 175.)

detailed mechanism for hydrolysis is known and can be described in three stages. Figure 2-15 shows how the disaccharide unit is hydrolyzed. The active site contains two amino acids, GLU and ASP, whose carboxylate groups participate in the hydrolysis. Initially, a proton ($H^+$ from the GLU) breaks the bond by binding to the oxygen between the two sugar rings, leaving an unbound, positively charged carbonium ion (carbon 4) in the right-hand sugar ring. This carbonium ion is temporarily stabilized by the negative charge on ASP above it (Figure 2-15 A, B). Then, a nearby water molecule ionizes and donates its proton to the negatively charged GLU while the hydroxy group (—OH) binds to the carbonium ion, and the reaction is complete (Figure 2-15 B, C). At completion, the original forms of the enzyme are regenerated and the hydrolyzed (split) chains of the peptidoglycan leave the active site of the enzyme. Once the peptidoglycan cover is split open (hydrolyzed) by lysozyme, the bacterium is no longer able to contain its high internal

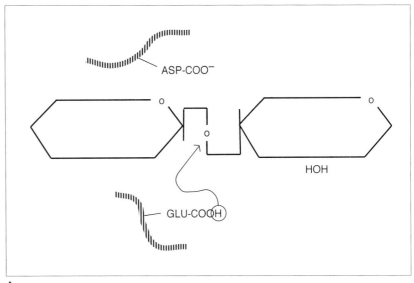

A

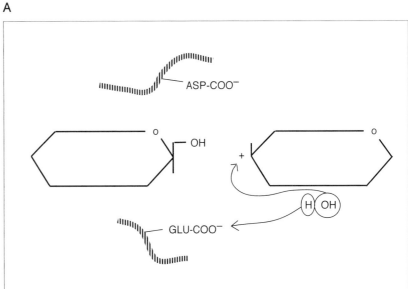

B

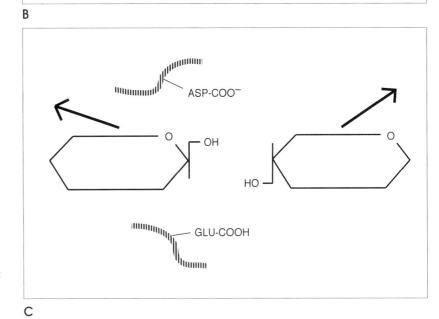

C

**FIGURE 2-15   The molecular mechanism of lysozyme catalysis.**
In order to break a glycosidic bond, the catalytic mechanism of lysozyme makes use of a nearby water molecule as well as two amino acids (asp and glu) located at the catalytic site. See the text for more information. (Adapted from Stryer L. *Biochemistry,* 3rd ed. New York: WH Freeman, 1988; 208.)

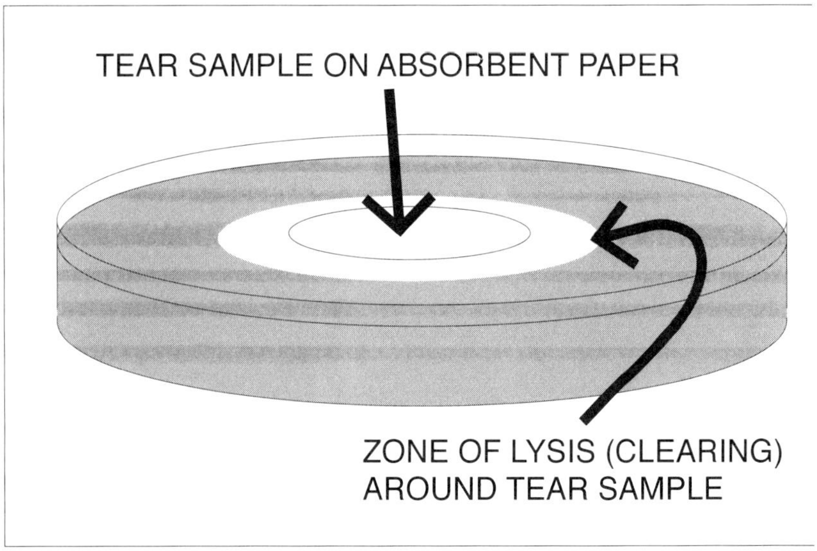

TEAR SAMPLE ON ABSORBENT PAPER

ZONE OF LYSIS (CLEARING)
AROUND TEAR SAMPLE

FIGURE 2-16   Quantitative Schirmer 1 test.
The tear sample containing lysozyme clears an area (zone of lysis) in an agar base (a gelatin-like product of seaweed) containing a standard amount of the bacterium *Micrococcus lysodeiticus*. The amount of lysozyme is proportional to the area cleared.

osmotic pressure with its plasma membrane alone, and it bursts open. Other protein components of tear film have been implicated in bactericidal action, but none are as efficient as lysozyme (Selsted and Martinez, 1982).

In addition to its bactericidal activity, lysozyme also serves as an important analytical indicator of tear dysfunction. Measurement of lysosome activity reflects the productivity of the main and accessory lacrimal glands (Gillette et al., 1981) as well as the status of aqueous deficiency of the tear film (van Bijsterveld and Westers, 1980). In the application of a quantitative Schirmer 1 test, for example, tear film is collected on filter paper discs and placed on a dish with agar containing $5 \times 10^7$ organisms of *Micrococcus lysodeiticus*. The lysozyme in the tear sample is allowed to hydrolyze the peptidoglycans and destroy the bacteria for 24 hours at 37°C. Then the diameter of the clear area of agar (i.e., destroyed bacteria) surrounding the tear sample is carefully measured (Figure 2-16). Typically, the diameter around samples from normal healthy persons is 19 to 30 mm, whereas the diameter around patients with keratoconjunctivitis sicca (dry eye) is 23 mm. The overlapped areas between healthy persons and patients who have dry eye account for only a 1% margin of error in making a diagnosis.

## Sodium, Potassium-Activated ATPase

Sodium, potassium-activated ATPase (Na, K-ATPase) is an enzyme in the plasma membranes of a wide variety of cells, but in ocular tissues it has two special functions: control of corneal hydration and production of aqueous fluid. The enzyme is membrane bound, which is to say that it is an integral protein that spans the width of cell plasma membranes. Its minimal quaternary structure is widely postulated to consist of four polypeptide chains, two $\alpha$- and two $\beta$-chains (Figure 2-17).

The $\alpha$-chains are the actual catalytic molecules for which the substrate is the high-energy compound ATP (see Chapter 3). The actual reaction is

$$ATP \xrightarrow{\text{ATPase}} ADP + P_i$$

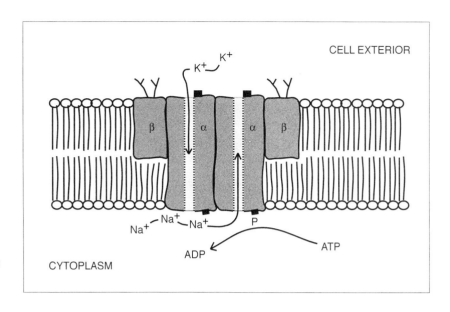

**FIGURE 2-17** Diagram of Na, K-ATPase incorporated in the plasma membrane of a cell.

The two α-subunits catalyze the transport of two K$^+$ ions inward and three Na$^+$ ions outward. The two dark rectangles on the cytoplasmic side are binding sites for phosphate and supply energy to drive the transport of these ions. The phosphate is obtained from the hydrolysis of ATP to ADP, which is the true catalytic event of this enzyme reaction. The two dark rectangles on the cell's exterior are binding sites for a cardiac glycoside known as ouabain (an inhibitor of this enzyme). The two β-subunits containing carbohydrate portions (the branchlike structures projecting into the cell's exterior) are thought to be necessary to stabilize and orient the α-subunits.

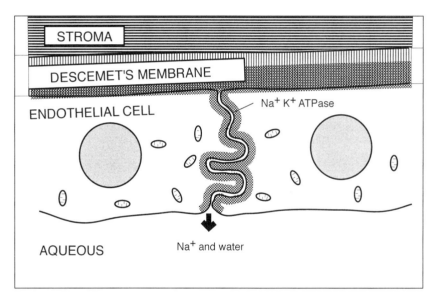

**FIGURE 2-18** Diagram of the endothelial cell (posterior) side of the cornea.

The location of Na, K-ATPase along the basolateral portions of the endothelial cells is indicated by wide gray lines. Sodium ions are believed to be pumped from the space between these cells to effect removal of excess water from the cornea.

However, there is more to this than what is described in the formula. Inorganic phosphate (P$_i$) becomes bound to one of the α-subunits and in the process supplies the energy necessary to transport three sodium ions out of a cell and two potassium ions inward. The exact detailed mechanism remains elusive, but investigators postulate that this may take place either by a conformational shuttle of the α-subunits or by the existence of holes or pores in the subunits through which the ions are pumped. In the control of corneal hydration (known as *deturgescence,* or literally, *declouding*), excess water is kept from entering the corneal stroma by the net flow of sodium ions pumped into the narrow channel (200 Å wide; Hogan et al., 1971) between adjacent endothelial cells. That is to say, that Na, k-ATPase pumps sodium ions into the channel, where they flow into the anterior chamber following the path of least resistance (diffusion). Water follows the sodium ions as an osmotic function (Figure 2-18).

It is reasonable to postulate ionic flow in this direction, since a higher density of trapped ions already exists in Descemet's membrane and beyond in the stroma. If the pumping mechanism did not exist, Na$^+$ ions and water

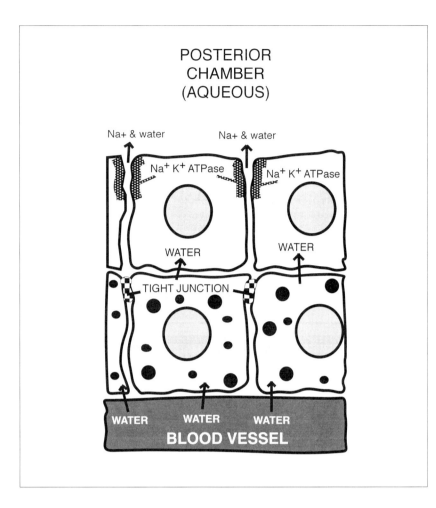

**FIGURE 2-19**    Diagram of the ciliary body showing nonpigmented (*top*) and pigmented (*bottom*) epithelial cells.

Na, K-ATPase is located on the basolateral membranes of the nonpigmented cells (dark gray portions), where the enzyme pumps excess $Na^+$ ions into the posterior chamber. Water flows from the adjacent blood vessels through the pigmented and nonpigmented cells and into the posterior chamber as a result of the osmotic gradient made by this flow of $Na^+$ ions. The tight junctions between pigmented cells represent a barrier to molecules larger than 20 Å. Water flows freely through the cell membranes and barriers when osmotically directed.

would continuously enter the central cornea, causing it to swell and become opaque. A similar mechanism is thought to operate in the nonpigmented epithelial cells of the ciliary body (Figure 2-19). In that case, a surplus of $Na^+$ ions is pumped into the posterior aqueous chamber by Na, K-ATPase and, in causing water to flow into the chamber osmotically, generates an intraocular pressure (Davson, 1990). Bicarbonate ions have also been postulated to contribute to these mechanisms, but the manner in which this occurs is a matter of speculation.

## Lactate Dehydrogenase

During the metabolism of carbohydrates (sugars) for the production of cellular energy, a point is reached at which the carbohydrate metabolite will be further processed either aerobically or anaerobically. The aerobic process (or pathway) has the advantage of producing energy efficiently (with high yield), whereas the anaerobic pathway has the advantage of producing energy very quickly and without oxygen, but inefficiently (i.e., many sugar molecules are required). Cells, ocular and nonocular, use both pathways. In particular, the corneal epithelium (especially when contact lenses are worn) and lens fiber cells (which normally are distant from nourishing blood vessels) make use of considerable fractions of anaerobic sugar metabolism. Surprisingly, photoreceptor cells also process a considerable fraction of sugar metabolites along the anaerobic pathway, and that process is actually dependent on oxygen. However, that takes place simply because the

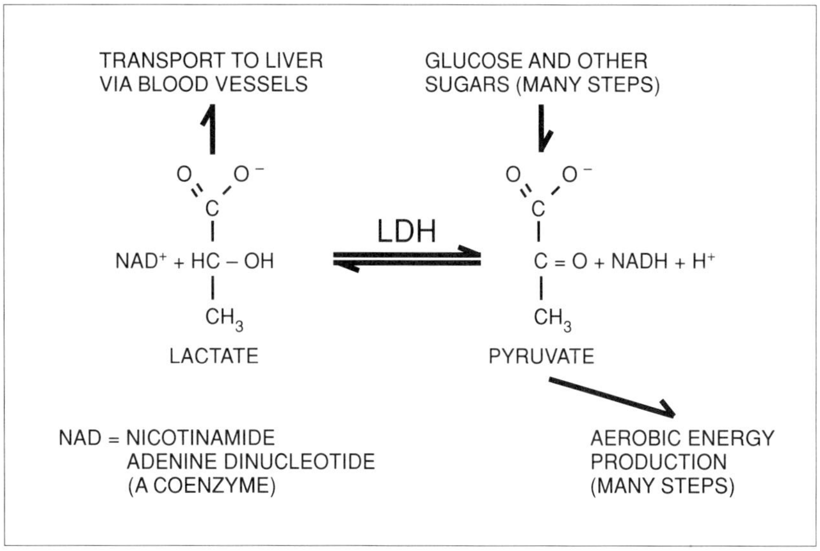

**FIGURE 2-20  Metabolic junction of carbohydrate metabolism between aerobic and nonaerobic pathways.**
At the top right, glucose and other carbohydrates are converted to pyruvate through many enzymatic reactions (see Chapter 3). If pyruvate is to be converted to cellular energy aerobically, it proceeds along the pathway at lower right. If pyruvate is to be shunted into the anaerobic pathway, the enzyme lactate dehydrogenase (LDH) catalyzes the reduction (gain of electrons) of pyruvate to form lactate. NADH (see text) is a cosubstrate for the reaction. The lactate formed is transported ultimately to the liver. The double arrow indicates that the reaction may proceed in both directions and is governed by the amount of pyruvate and lactate present.

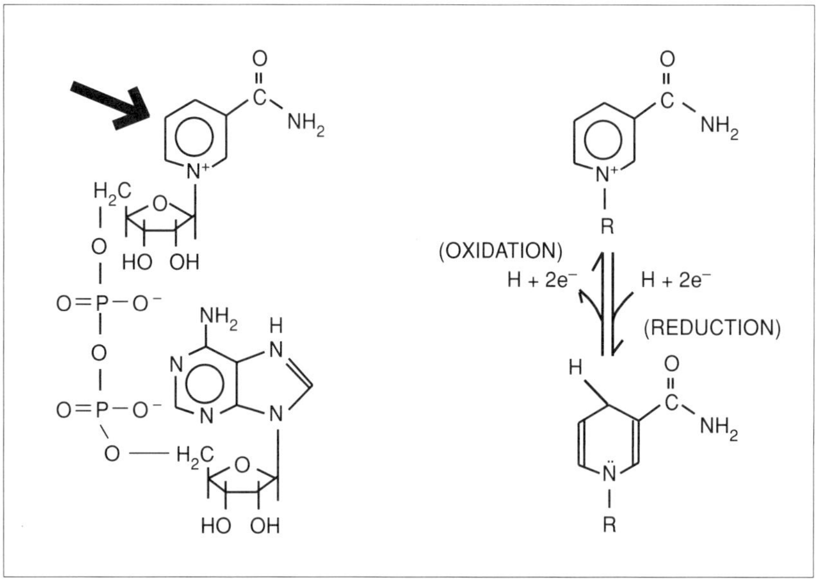

**FIGURE 2-21  A molecule of nicotinamide adenine dinucleotide (NAD⁺) in the oxidized state (left).**
The nicotinamide ring portion (arrow) is the site of electron gain (reduction) or loss (oxidation). In fact, both a hydrogen atom (H) and two electrons (e⁻) are transferred to and from the nicotinamide ring, as shown on the right-hand side of the diagram. Oxidation-reduction mechanisms similar to this are common for many of the coenzymes derived from the water-soluble vitamins.

photoreceptor's high rate of metabolism overloads the aerobic pathway. Photoreceptors are strongly bent on obtaining energy in any way possible to maintain their primary function of visual transduction.

The enzyme that operates at the metabolic junction of aerobic and anaerobic metabolism is *lactate dehydrogenase,* and is found in the cytoplasm of all eukaryotic cells. The reaction is diagrammed in Figure 2-20. Pyruvate, the metabolic substrate for the reaction, is formed from dietary carbohydrates such as glucose, fructose, and galactose. A second substrate, the coenzyme nicotinamide adenine dinucleotide (reduced) or NADH, provides electrons for the reduction of pyruvate to lactate (Figure 2-21). NADH is one of a number of coenzymes that are metabolically derived from water-soluble vitamins (Table 2-1). The enzyme itself (Figure 2-22), abbreviated here as LDH, is a protein tetramer (i.e., four polypeptide chains) with a total molecular weight of 140 kd.

This enzyme has at least three different kinds of polypeptides that may occur in various combinations of tetramers. They are designated H (for

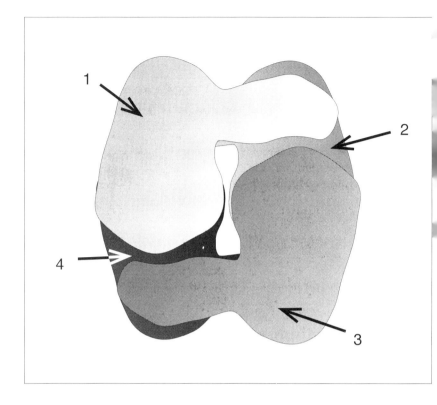

**FIGURE 2-22   The quaternary structure of lactate dehydrogenase.**
Each numbered subunit is indicated by a different shade of grey, and each possesses a catalytic site. Adapted from Cantos CR, and Schimmel PR. *Biophysical Chemistry. Part 1. The Conformation of Biological Macromolecules.* San Francisco: WH Freeman, 1980; 120, 124.

**TABLE 2-1   Some Coenzymes and Their Water-Soluble Vitamin Sources**

| Coenzyme* | Related Vitamin | Functions |
|---|---|---|
| NAD<br>NADP | Niacin | Oxidation-reduction reactions in carbohydrate metabolism |
| FAD<br>TPP<br>PP | Riboflavin ($B_2$)<br>Thiamine ($B_1$)<br>Pyridoxal ($B_6$) | Oxidation-reduction metabolism in mitochondria |
| DAC | Cobalamin ($B_{12}$) | Methionine synthesis, fatty acid degradation |
| Ascorbate | Ascorbic acid (C) | Oxidation-reduction of toxic substances |

*Key: NAD, nicotinamide adenine dinucleotide; NADP, nicotinamide adenine dinucleotide phosphate; FAD, flavine adenine dinucleotide; TPP, thiamine pyrophosphate; PP, pyridoxal phosphate; DAC, deoxyadenosyl cobalamin.

heart), M (muscle), and K (a designation first applied to the polypeptide found in cancer cells). Various combinations of these polypeptides can "customize" the activity of LDH: $H_4$ (found in heart, of course), $M_4$ (for the muscle cell enzyme) as well as $H_3M$, $H_2M_2$, and $HM_3$ found in other cell types. The $K_4$ or $LDH_K$ type is found in photoreceptors as well as cancer cells and is characteristic of cells that have a high metabolic rate. Different forms of a single enzyme are known as *isozymes*. A more recent term, "isoform," has the same meaning. This distinction is important in ocular tissues, inasmuch as the kinetic properties of each enzyme type determine (1) the relative proportions of aerobic and anaerobic pathways used by the cells and (2) whether the cell will obtain energy quickly (anaerobic metabolism) or cheaply (aerobic metabolism). One would find, therefore, that with the $H_4$ LDH enzyme:

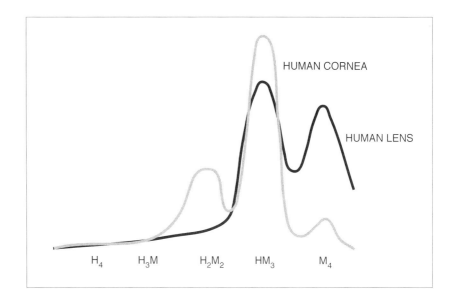

**FIGURE 2-23    Density pattern of the isozyme forms of LDH in human cornea and lens.**
Both tissues are oriented toward a predominance of anaerobic metabolism, but with more flexibility in the cornea. (Adapted from Jacq C, Liotet S, Warnet VN, and Anata M. Lactic dehydrogenase isozymes in the ocular tissues and liquids. *Ophthalmol Basel* 1982;184:174–178.)

$$\text{Lactate} \longrightarrow \text{Pyruvate}$$
$$\frac{[\text{Pyruvate}]}{[\text{Lactate}]} = K_{eq} > 1$$

In this case, lactate formation is impeded and pyruvate is retained.

The $M_4$ LDH would permit the reaction to proceed equally in either direction. Here, the formation of lactate is driven by the concentration of pyruvate:

$$\text{Lactate} \rightleftharpoons \text{Pyruvate}$$
$$\frac{[\text{Pyruvate}]}{[\text{Lactate}]} = K_{eq} = 1$$

The K form of LDH is one whose catalytic rate increases with the partial pressure of oxygen ($pO_2$). One might say that $K_{eq}$ approaches 1 as the $pO_2$ increases.

In the corneal epithelium it is important that the cells be able to survive under conditions of relatively low $pO_2$ as occurs with lid closure and, even more so, with contact lens wear when oxygen transmissibility through the contact lens is impeded. Under such conditions, epithelial cells, which normally obtain oxygen from the precorneal tear film, must shunt their carbohydrate metabolism to lactate production via LDH. This mechanism can successfully support epithelial cells down to $pO_2$ values as low as 15 to 20 mm Hg. It is known that in rabbit cornea the synthesis of lactate increases at lowered pressures of about 15 to 20 mm Hg. Even in isolated rabbit corneas, the synthesis of lactate increases about 33% when atmospheric air is entirely replaced by nitrogen. Jacq et al. (1982) found that the relative proportion of isozymes of LDH in isolated whole human cornea was 25% $H_2M_2$, 65% $HM_3$, and 10% $M_4$ (Figure 2-23). These types would favor lactate production under conditions of oxygen starvation.

In the whole lens, the dominant population of cells is lens fiber cells, whose metabolic rate is low compared to that of most cell types. Considering that the lens is also rather isolated from its blood supply and that the deeper lens fiber cells have no subcellular organelles, it is not surprising that these cells make little use of oxygen for metabolism. Jacq et al. (1982) found only $HM_3$ and $M_4$ LDH isozymes in whole human lenses (see Figure 2-23).

In the retina, $LDH_K$ acts to open the pathway to lactate, to aid rapid metabolism of glucose, since the energy demand in photoreceptors is very high. Saavedra et al. (1985) described this enzyme form as being quite different from the other common isozymes of LDH. In 1988, Li et al. found that $LDH_K$ was actually LDH $M_4$ modified in two ways: phosphate is present on tyrosine residue No. 238 near the active site (causing a conformational change), and the enzyme is complexed with other proteins. Either or both of these changes may explain its sensitivity to oxygen. The production of lactate in retina is higher than in any other aerobic tissue, and the phenomenon of high lactate production, coupled with high glucose and oxygen consumption, has been termed *the Warburg effect* (Warburg, 1924).

## Aldose Reductase

Another enzyme linked to the metabolism of carbohydrates is aldose reductase. Although the catalytic activity of this enzyme is not related to normal carbohydrate metabolism, its function has been shown to cause cataracts in persons who have either diabetes or galactosemia. The enzyme belongs to a family of enzymes called aldo-ketoreductases (Flynn, 1986). Kador et al. (1986) describe the enzyme as having a molecular weight range of 28 to 45 kd depending on the source but it has only a single polypeptide chain. It is postulated to exist in globular form, like many water-soluble enzymes. The biochemical activity of aldose reductase was discovered by the work of van Heyningen (1959) and Kinoshita (1965, 1974). Aldose reductase catalyzes the following reactions in the lens:

Note that both reactions require the coenzyme NADPH.

These reactions are the first step of a two-step pathway, known as the *polyol pathway*. The intermediate products sorbitol and galactitol are polyols, or polyhydroxy-alcohols. The connection to cataract formation is the fact that these polyols produce an osmotic imbalance in lens fiber cells, causing them to swell and, eventually to burst. The cataract is represented by the light-scattering produced by the cellular debris. Normally the enzyme is inactive or nearly so until the concentration of either glucose or galactose in

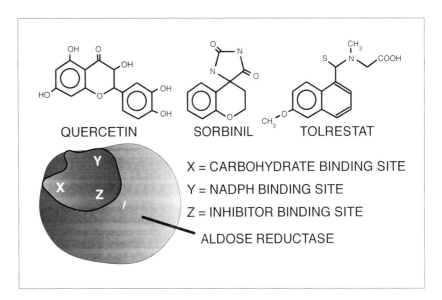

QUERCETIN        SORBINIL        TOLRESTAT

X = CARBOHYDRATE BINDING SITE

Y = NADPH BINDING SITE

Z = INHIBITOR BINDING SITE

ALDOSE REDUCTASE

**FIGURE 2-24**   This diagram of aldose reductase indicates the location of separate regions for carbohydrate, NADPH, and inhibitor-binding sites. On the top are some typical inhibitors that have been tried for this enzyme. Note that all are ring structures with considerable hydrophobicity.

the lens rises. This occurs, of course, in the diseases associated with these carbohydrates (see Chapter 3). Since the $K_m$ for glucose is 100 mM for aldose reductase and since fasting blood levels are normally about 5 mM, the enzyme's activity is virtually nil. Even after a meal, when the blood sugar level may rise temporarily to 10 mM, the enzyme is minimally activated. In diabetes, however, blood sugar levels can approach or exceed 20 mM for sustained periods if uncontrolled. This brings about activation of aldose reductase.

Much interest has been focused on the development of a therapeutic inhibitor of aldose reductase, not only as an anticataractic agent but also for possible prevention of diabetic retinopathy due to aldose reductase. Kador et al. (1986) explained that there is an inhibitor site on the enzyme that is lipophilic (or hydrophobic) and is, therefore, capable of associating with a wide variety of fat-soluble substances that may act as inhibitors. Binding sites for the sugar, NADPH, and inhibitor are in separate locations (Figure 2-24). The structures of three of the many inhibitors tried are shown— quercetin, sorbinil, and tolrestat. Quercetin was studied earlier as an inhibitor, but was found to be too weak. Sorbinil has undergone extensive testing, but unfortunately the occurrence of hypersensitivity reactions is unacceptably high (Frank, 1990). Tolrestat is a newer agent whose efficacy has not yet been determined (Frank, 1990). Inhibition of aldose reductase is considered to be either uncompetitive or noncompetitive (Figure 2-25), according to investigations made by Bhatnagar et al. (1990). The mechanism depends on the inhibitor that is used.

## Summary

Enzymes are proteins which act as biological catalysts for a variety of cellular and extracellular reactions. In the eye, enzymes promote many of the same reactions that occur in other parts of the body, but some have specialized functions. Lysozyme acts in the precorneal tear film to destroy Gram-positive bacteria by hydrolysis of their peptidoglycan coats. The enzyme may also be used to verify normal tear production. Na, K-ATPase acts in the corneal endothelium to maintain a normal rate of deturgescence. The same enzyme also generates the intraocular pressure originating in the ciliary

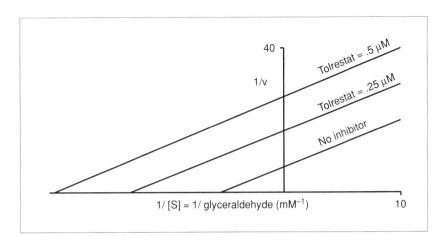

**FIGURE 2-25** Lineweaver-Burk graph of uncompetitive inhibition of aldose reductase with the inhibitor tolrestat. Compare this diagram with Figure 2-9, bottom. The substrate used in this case was glyceraldehyde (a simple sugar). The unit 10 on the *x*-axis stands for millimolar (M) concentration. The unit 40 on the *y*-axis stands for milimoles per liter converted to product per minute. Both units are reciprocal units.

body. Both functions are the result of enzymatic cation pumping and the generation of osmotic flow. Lactate dehydrogenase is an enzyme involved in shunting carbohydrate metabolites between aerobic and anaerobic metabolism. This is accomplished by having the enzyme exist in several forms (isozymes). A special isozyme in the retina promotes maximal production of cellular energy. Aldose reductase is a lens enzyme that is normally inactive, but in persons with either diabetes and or galactosemia it catalyzes the formation of polyols, which bring about the osmotic destruction of lens fiber cells. Considerable effort has been made to develop an inhibitor for this enzyme.

## References

Bhatnagar A, Liu S, Das B, Ansari NH, and Srivastava SK. Inhibition kinetics of human kidney aldose and aldehyde reductases by aldose reductase inhibitors. *Biochem Pharm* 1990;39:1115–1124.

Davson H. *Physiology of the Eye*, 5th ed. New York: Pergamon, 1990;32-36.

Flynn TG. Aldose and aldehyde reductase in animal tissues. *Metabolism* 1986;35(Suppl 1):105–108.

Frank RN. Aldose reductase inhibition. The chemical key to the control of diabetic retinopathy? *Arch Ophthalmol* 1990;108:1229–1231.

Gillette TE, Greiner JV, and Allansmith MR. Immunohistochemical localization of human tear lysozyme. *Arch Ophthalmol* 1981;99:298–300.

Hogan MJ, Alvarado JA, and Weddell JE. *Histology of the Human Eye.* Philadelphia: W.B. Saunders, 1971;55–111.

Jacq C, Liotet S, Warnet VN, and Arrata M. Lactic dehydrogenase isozymes in the ocular tissues and liquids. *Ophthalmol Basel* 1982;184:174–178.

Kador PF, Kinoshita JH, and Sharpless NE. The aldose reductase inhibitor site. *Metabolism* 1986;35 (Suppl 1):109–113.

Kinoshita JH. Cataracts in galactosemia. *Invest Ophthalmol* 1965; 5: 786–789.

Kinoshita JH. Mechanisms initiating cataract formation. *Invest Ophthalmol* 1974;13:713–724.

Li SS-L, Pan Y-CE, Sharief FS, Evans MJ, Lin M-F, Clinton GM, and Holbrook JJ. Cancer-associated lactate dehydrogenase is a tyrosylphosphorylated form of human LDH-M, a skeletal muscle isozyme. *Cancer Invest* 1988;6:93–101.

Mathews CK, and van Holde KE. *Biochemistry.* Redwood City, Calif.: Benjamin/Cummings, 1990;360–361.

Palmer T. *Understanding Enzymes.* New York: John Wiley & Sons, 1981;119–124.

Saavedra RA, Cordoba C, and Anderson GR. LDHk in the retina of diverse vertebrate species: A possible link to the Warburg effect. *Exp Eye Res* 1985;41:365–370.

Selsted ME, and Martinez RJ. Isolation and purification of bacteriocides from human tears. Exp Eye Res 1982:34:305–318.

Sen DK, and Sarin GS. Immunoassay of human tear film lysozyme. *Am J. Ophthalmol* 1980;90:715–718.

Stryer L. *Biochemistry,* 3rd ed. New York: WH Freeman, 1988;201–202.

van Bijsterveld OP, and Westers JC. Therapie bei Keratokonjunktivitis sicca. *Klin Monatsbl Augenheilkd* 1980;177:52–57.

van Heyningen R. Formation of polyols by the lens of the rat with 'sugar' cataract. *Nature* 1959;184:194–195.

Warburg O, Posener K, and Negalein E. Uber den Stoffwechsel de Carcinonzelle. *Biochem Z* 1924;152:308–344.

Whikehart DR, Montgomery B, and Hafer LM. Sodium and potassium saturation kinetics of $Na^+K^+$ATPase in plasma membranes from corneal endothelium: Fresh tissue vs. tissue culture. *Curr Eye Res* 1987;6:709–717.

# Chapter 3

# Carbohydrates

## Review of Structures and Properties

Sweet-tasting substances have been known since ancient times. However, sugars were not isolated as chemical substances until the 18th and 19th centuries (Roehrig, 1984). For example, one of the most common sugars, glucose, was isolated by Dumas in 1838 from the hydrolysis of starch. The structures of glucose and other sugars were determined by Emil Fischer just after the turn of the century. The name "sugar," which is Arabic in origin, is replaced in biochemistry by the term "carbohydrate," literally a compound of *carbon* and *water* having the general formula $C_n(H_2O)_n$. Carbohydrates are more properly classified as polyhydroxy compounds, which may contain either aldehydes, ketones, alcohols, acids, or amines as well as their derivatives. The simplest carbohydrates, which are used for cellular food or fuel, are either aldehydes or ketones; other types usually serve to support tissue morphology (form) (Figure 3-1).

Carbohydrate structure may be represented in three ways called: Fischer, Haworth, and conformational (Figure 3-2). The Haworth structure represents a reasonable compromise between the misleading *Fischer structure* and the somewhat confusing (but accurate) *conformational structure*. The Haworth structure is used in the remainder of this book. In these figures it should be understood that the heavier lines are closest to the reader. Hydrogen atoms are implied at the end of each vertical line, and the carbons within the ring are not written.

Carbohydrates are capable of extensive isomerization, either on their own or by the action of cellular enzymes. In the case of glucose (and other simple carbohydrates) C-1 can form an oxygen bridge by itself with C-5 to construct either a six-membered closed structure known as a *pyran ring* or a five-membered closed ring known as a *furan ring*. This it does about 99% of the time while in solution (Figure 3-3). C-1 is also known as the *reducing carbon*, since it can donate electrons to other substances. This property has served as the basis for determining the concentration of glucose in blood

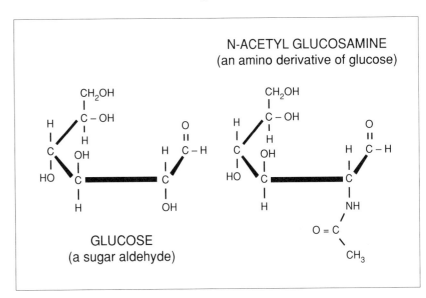

**FIGURE 3-1  Two examples of carbohydrates, glucose and *N*-acetyl glucosamine.**
Note that both have an aldehyde group and multiple hydroxy groups. The latter characteristic increases their water solubility. *N*-acetylglucosamine is metabolically derived from glucose.

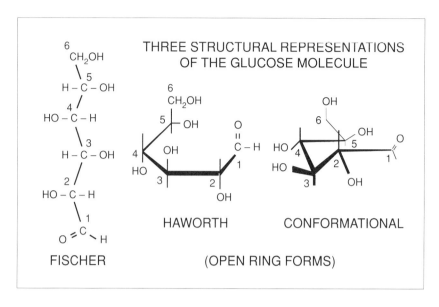

**FIGURE 3-2    Representations of the glucose molecule.**
The Haworth structure is a commonly used representation for carbohydrates, though the conformational structure is more accurate. The use of the latter structure makes it difficult to distinguish individual carbohydrate types in three-dimensional representation. The Fischer structure is the least accurate of the three representations. Carbons are numbered 1 through 6.

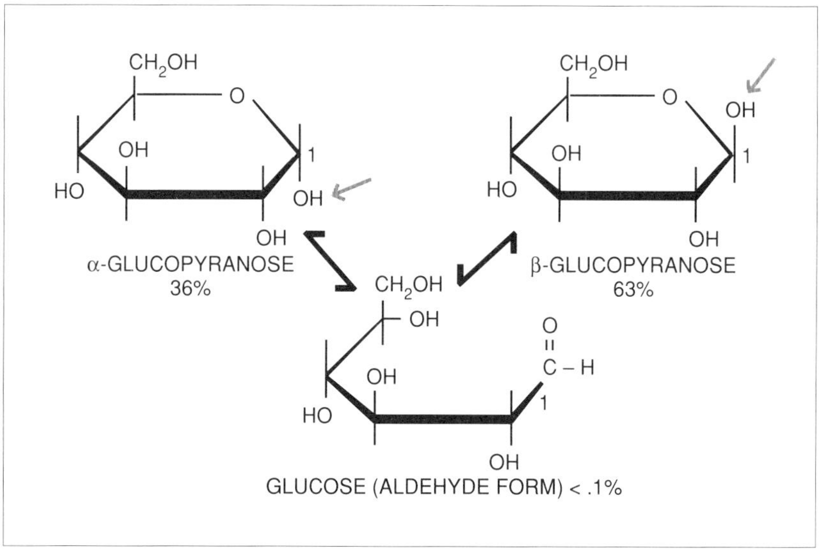

**FIGURE 3-3    Isomeric forms of glucose in solution.**
Monosaccharides constantly alternate their isomeric forms by opening and closing their ring structures. The percentages indicate which forms are present at any given time. By convention, when the hydroxy group on C-1 is down (in the figure), the isomer is designated as the α-form and when it is up, it is the β-form.

and urine. For example, the aldehyde of C-1 reacts with o-toluidine to form a colored covalent complex that gives a reliable estimate of glucose concentrations (Caraway and Watts, 1986) (Figure 3-4). It has also been discovered that C-1 can react with proteins to form a permanent bond when present in high concentrations, as occurs in diabetes (Cohen, 1986).

The most common six- and five-member ringed carbohydrates of biological importance are glucose, galactose, mannose, and fructose. These carbohydrates are called: monosaccharides (from the Greek *monos,* [single], and sakcharon, sugar). They consist of a unit or single ring (Figure 3-5). All four carbohydrates have nutritional value for cells, but glucose is the most important.

Two-sugar units are also quite common. They are called: *disaccharides* (literally: two sugars). Some of these are: maltose, sucrose, and lactose. Maltose is a disaccharide that occurs as the result of the hydrolysis of starch (a sugar polymer described later) and that can be found in germinating cereals and grains. It consists of two glucose units held together by an oxygen bridge (Figure 3-6). *Sucrose,* common table sugar, comes from a variety of

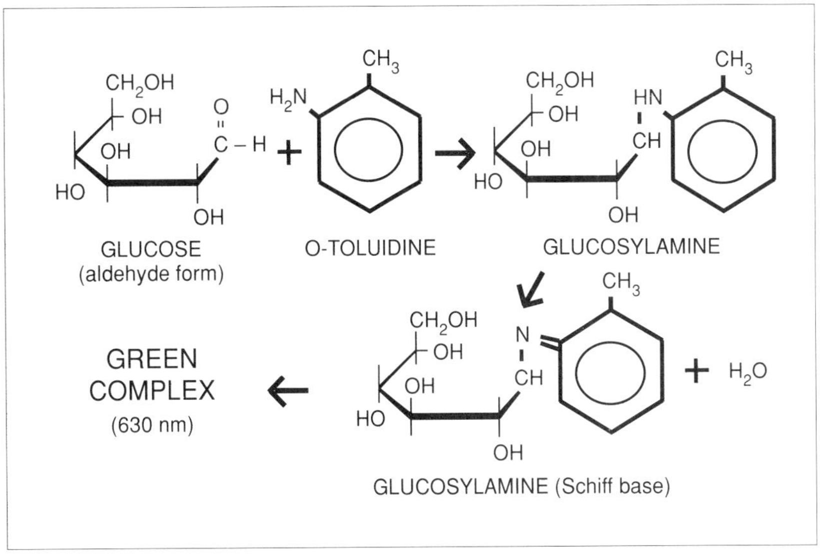

**FIGURE 3-4   Reaction of glucose with o-toluidine.**
A common laboratory procedure (one of several) for determining the concentration of glucose in blood and other body fluids is the *o*-toluidine method. *Ortho*-toluidine forms a Schiff base with glucose (as a glucosylamine). Subsequently, the glucosylamine reacts to produce a green complex of undetermined structure (Caraway and Watts, 1986) that is proportional to the glucose concentration and may be read in a spectrophotometer at 630 nm.

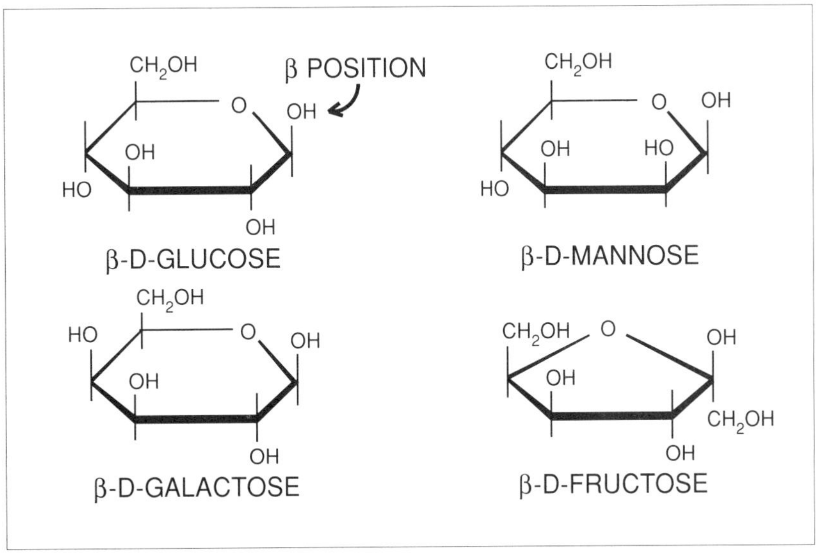

**FIGURE 3-5   Structures of four common nutritional monosaccharides.**
These monosaccharides are used as sources of ATP and for synthesizing building blocks of extracellular polymers (after metabolic processing).

plants, cane, beets, pineapple, and carrots among them. It is composed of one glucose and one fructose molecule also joined by an oxygen bridge (see Figure 3-6). *Lactose,* the disaccharide in milk, is made up of galactose and glucose with an oxygen bridge. The nature of the oxygen bridge in disaccharides varies. In maltose it is known as an $\alpha$ (1→4) linkage meaning that it joins C-1 of the left-hand unit to C-4 of the right-hand unit and that the position of the oxygen joining C-1 is $\alpha$ (down) relative to the carbon. In sucrose the linkage is an ($\alpha$ 1→2) type, but the fructose unit is flipped over so that what appears to be C-5 is actually C-2. In lactose the linkage is a ($\beta$ 1→4) type. That is, the oxygen linkage is $\beta$ (up) to C-1 on the galactose. In disaccharides, only the right-hand carbohydrate (see Figure 3-6) may have a reactive or reducing carbon.

Carbohydrates that have more than two units are known as either *oligosaccharides* (a few sugars) or *polysaccharides* (many sugars), depending on their chain length. The division is arbitrary, but when the number of saccharide units is greater than 10, "polysaccharide" is the preferred term (Roehrig, 1984).

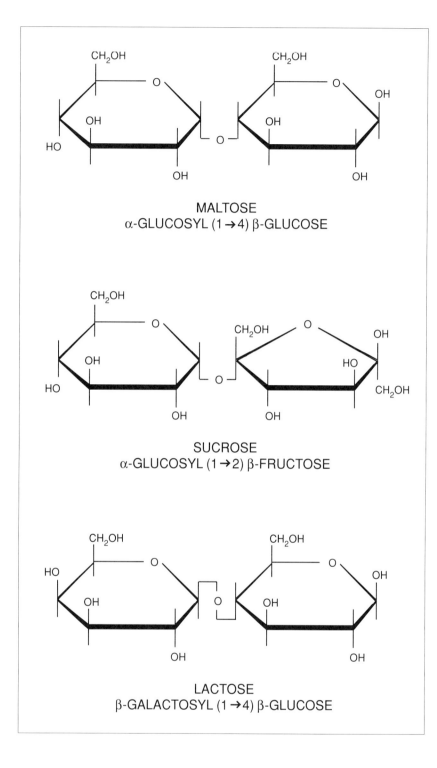

**FIGURE 3-6   Three disaccharides common in the human diet.**
Maltose is a hydrolysis product of starch, whereas sucrose is common table sugar.

Polysaccharides serve two principal functions in all biological tissues, a storage function and a structural (morphological) function. Storage polysaccharides in animal tissues have a greater diversity of branching linkages than those in plants. The form in animals is known as *glycogen* and the two common forms in plants are amylose and amylopectin (collectively called *starch*). The straight and branching linkages are shown in Figure 3-7. The extensive branching of glycogen causes the molecule to be very compact, which is highly desirable for storage purposes. Glycogen is stored in the cytoplasm of cells and is a very large molecule with a typical molecular

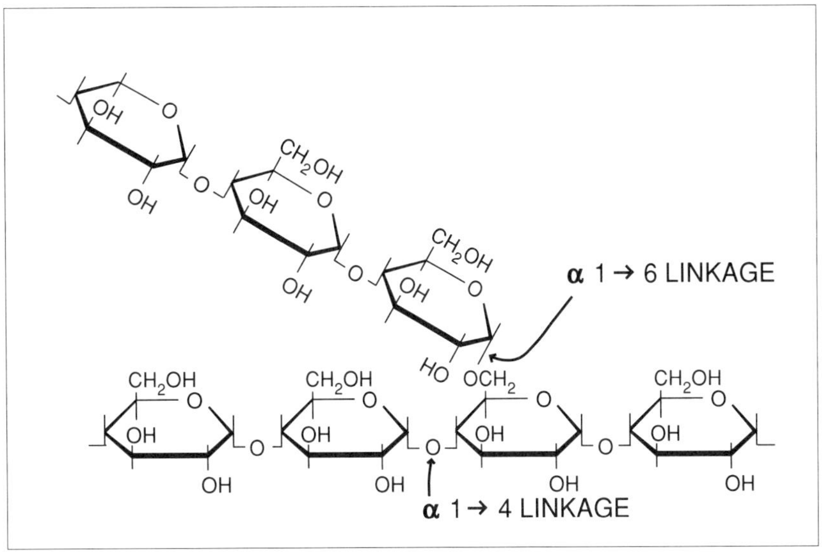

**FIGURE 3-7    Partial structure and bonds of storage forms of carbohydrates in animal and plant cells.**
All forms have glucose molecules linked in ($\alpha$1→4) bonds. Glycogen (in animals) also has ($\alpha$1→6) bonds (branches), which occur as frequently as every fourth carbohydrate. Amylopectin (in plants) has ($\alpha$1→6) branches less frequently than glycogen. Amylose (also in plants) has no ($\alpha$1→6) branches.

weight of several thousand kilodaltons (Stryer, 1988). In the eye, some tissues have cells that are known to maintain glycogen stores, the corneal epithelial cells and the retinal Müller cells in particular. Some ocular cells do not contain glycogen, such as corneal endothelial cells and retinal photoreceptors. The latter use glucose at such a high rate that they cannot store it. Structural polysaccharides will be considered in the section on glycosaminoglycans and oligosaccharides.

## Review of Metabolism

Carbohydrates play two principal roles in ocular and nonocular tissues: they support metabolism by acting as fuels and they are significant constituents of biological structures. In order to look at their role as fuels, it is necessary to consider the nature of metabolism, especially anabolic and catabolic processes. Anabolic processes in cells are the reactions that synthesize cellular components and maintain their functions. These reactions are coupled to catabolic processes that might be considered degradative, but actually provide energy for the cell to carry out its anabolic reactions (e.g., making proteins, building cell walls, causing visual transduction).

Instead of requiring heat energy (as a car does), cells use high-energy compounds to drive their synthetic (anabolic) reactions. The most important of these compounds is adenosine triphosphate (ATP). This compound (Figure 3-8) has three molecular parts: adenine, ribose, and three phosphate groups. The adenine and ribose portions act as "handles" to position the molecule at enzyme-reactive sites in order to release its potential energy by breaking, usually, the outermost phosphate bond. This action either "powers up" the enzyme for catalytic tasks or causes the transfer of that energy to some product of the reaction. Bridger and Henderson (1983) have stated that the potential energy in ATP stems from the crowded negative charges of the phosphate groups and the somewhat constricted ability of the electrons to move about (delocalize) within the phosphate groups. Carbohydrates act in cells to return relatively lower energy adenosine diphosphate (ADP) to its higher energy ATP form and maintain this cellular energy

**FIGURE 3-8   Adenosine triphosphate.**
Energy is released from ATP with the hydrolysis of each phosphate group. Usually, only the outermost phosphate is released to form ADP. The release of the outermost phosphate group transfers 31 kJ of energy under standard conditions (pH 7, 25°C). However, under actual conditions in cells that energy transfer may be estimated to be in the range of 50 kJ (Mathews and van Holde, 1990). For calorie counters, the equivalent amounts are 7.41 and 11.95 kilocalories respectively.

system. In fact, not only carbohydrates, but also lipids and proteins are capable of "making" ATP according to the following general metabolic scheme:

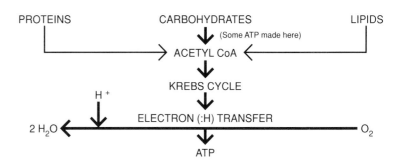

In the scheme, acetyl CoA is an intermediate two-carbon unit (acetate) coupled to a carrier molecule (coenzyme A). The two-carbon unit can be made from proteins and lipids as well as carbohydrates, but carbohydrates are the most common and immediate sources of acetyl CoA for ATP production. In fact, the use of proteins and lipids to make ATP can be pathological (destructive) to tissues when that use becomes excessive. This can occur in either diabetes mellitus or in starvation. The metabolic pathways, from carbohydrates to acetyl CoA through the Krebs cycle to ATP production, consist of series of biochemical reactions that are all enzyme catalyzed. The electron transfer, shown in the scheme, is caused by the Krebs cycle. It is explained further on.

The reactions may occur in the presence (aerobic metabolism) or absence (anaerobic metabolism) of oxygen. Up to the generation of acetyl CoA, all reactions take place in the cytoplasm of the cell. Beyond that stage they occur in the mitochondria. The storage of carbohydrates (as glycogen) as well as the synthesis of lipids (as fatty acids) and nucleic acids (as pentoses) and cell detoxification are also linked to these pathways. The pathways are outlined in Figure 3-9. All ocular cells, as well as other animal cells, make use of these pathways in varying degrees.

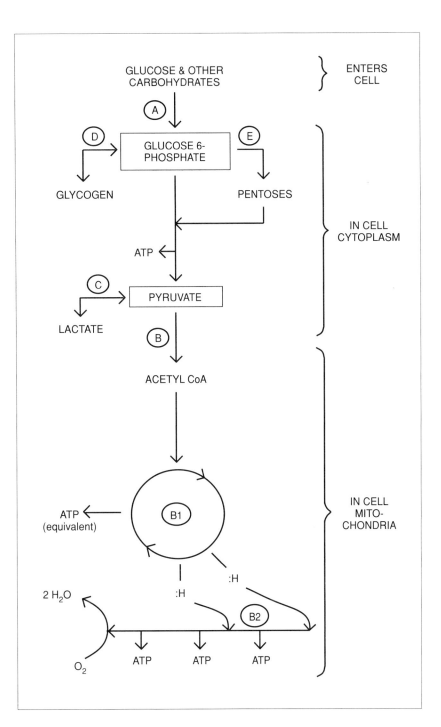

**FIGURE 3-9** Diagrammed outline of carbohydrate metabolism.

Glucose and other monosaccharides enter the pathways initially at the Embden-Meyerhof (EM) pathway (A). Glucose and galactose enter as glucose 6-phosphate, whereas fructose and mannose enter as fructose 6-phosphate (not shown here). All carbohydrates are enzymatically converted to the three-carbon triose pyruvate at the end of the E-M pathway. The process is also known as *glycolysis*. A small amount of ATP is produced in the formation of pyruvate. Some pyruvate is converted to acetyl CoA (B), and at this point the triose has entered the aerobic phase of glycolysis. This takes place in the cellular mitochondria. Acetyl CoA is incorporated (B1) into the Krebs cycle (also known as the tricarboxylic acid cycle or citric acid cycle). In the cycle, ATP equivalents (guanosine triphosophate [GTP]) and electron-bearing compounds (NADH, FADH₂) are released. The electron-bearing compounds are shuttled along the mitochondrial inner membrane (B2) in a process known as *oxidative phosphorylation*, which results indirectly in the production of substantial quantities of ATP. The electron transport eventually ends at the formation of water (by combining hydrogen and oxygen), while the Krebs cycle forms CO₂ (not shown), both as byproducts. Some pyruvate is converted to lactate (C), in which case the triose enters the anaerobic phase of glycolysis. Near the top of the scheme it can be seen that glucose 6-phosphate can also be converted to glycogen (D) for storage purposes or to pentoses (E) for other metabolic requirements of the cell. The boxed carbohydrate intermediates, are at metabolic crossroads.

## Glycolysis

When carbohydrates are consumed, whether as monosaccharides or in some chain form such as starch, they enter the circulation (after being converted enzymatically to monosaccharides as necessary) and travel from the gut to individual cells, which they enter. How they enter cells is considered on page 73. In the cellular cytoplasm, carbohydrates are immediately phosphorylated to prevent their escape from the cell. This is so, inasmuch as the negative charges on the phosphate group do not allow the carbohydrate to pass through the hydrophobic interior of the cell's plasma membrane. This is the first step of the Embden-Meyerhof (E-M) glycolytic pathway, and, ironically, requires a molecule of ATP (Figure 3-10). Glucose

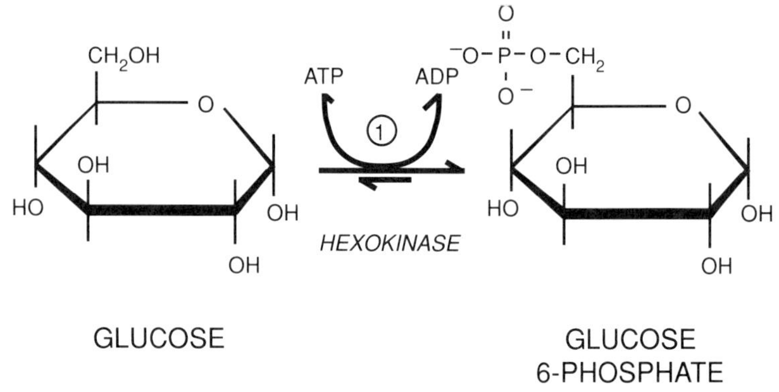

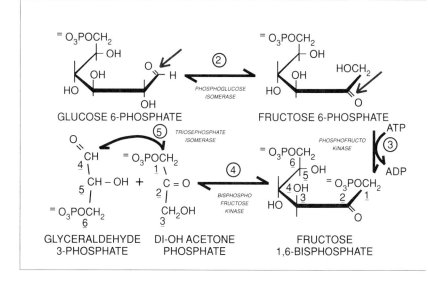

**FIGURE 3-10   The initial reaction of glycolysis.**
The purpose of the first step in glycolysis is to retain
carbohydrates within cells by adding a phosphate group.
The double negative charge at carbon 6 of glucose prevents
any diffusion through the cell membrane.

**FIGURE 3-11   Reactions 2 through 5 of the E-M pathway.**
Each reaction is numbered. The names of the enzymes are
given in italics. In reaction 4, the substrate and products
have their carbons numbered to show their positions before
and after the reaction.

6-phosphate represents a metabolic junction for the continuation of glycolysis, storage (as glycogen), or the pentose shunt (see Figure 3-9).

In subsequent steps of glycolysis, the carbohydrate is prepared for frac-
tionation into three-carbon units, split apart, and then further rearranged to
generate four new molecules of ATP. Figures 3-11 and 3-12 show the additional steps in these reactions. In Figure 3-11, glucose 6-phosphate (in its
open-chain, reactive form) is isomerized to fructose 6-phosphate. The
movement of the carbonyl group (*dotted arrows*) allows the molecule to be
phosphorylated at C-1 in the following step. This requires a second molecule
of ATP, and the reaction has energetically primed the molecule for splitting
(the actual step of glycolysis). In reaction 4, the phosphorylated carbohydrate
is broken into two three-carbon isomers. The presence of phosphate groups
on each ensures that they will remain within the cell cytoplasm. The isomers
can be interconverted due to the catalytic action of an isomerase enzyme. In
fact, virtually all of the dihydroxyacetone phosphate is converted to glyceraldehyde 3-phosphate while that compound is being funneled off into the remainder of the E-M pathway. In this manner the cell acquires two metabolic
intermediates from each carbohydrate it sends through the pathway.

Note (Figure 3-11, reaction 3) that conversion of fructose 6-phosphate to
fructose 1,6-bisphosphate is catalyzed by the enzyme phosphofructokinase.

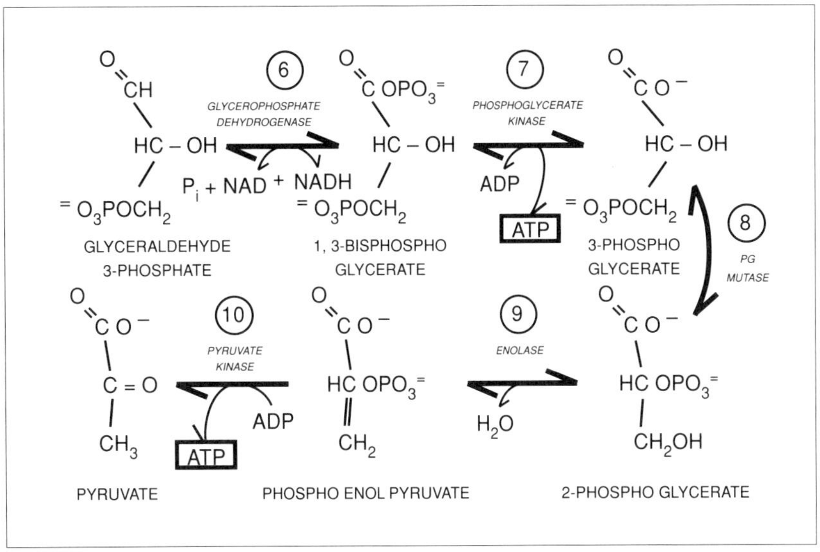

**FIGURE 3-12** Reactions 6 through 10 of the E-M pathway.
ATP molecules produced in reactions 7 and 10 are shown in boxes. See Figure 3-11.

This allosteric enzyme dominates by controlling the rate of the entire pathway. It is unidirectional, and its rate is influenced by the varying energy requirements of individual cells, which depend on such factors as the level of ATP (low levels stimulate it), hydrogen ion $H^+$ concentration (high levels inhibit it), and fructose 6-phosphate (high levels indirectly stimulate it) (Stryer, 1988).

In the remainder of the pathway (see Figure 3-12) phosphate groups are transferred to ADP to form ATP (reactions 7 and 10). In step 6, glyceraldehyde 3-phosphate acquires a second phosphate group. This time, however, it comes from inorganic phosphate in the cytoplasm rather than ATP. This reaction requires the coenzyme nicotinamide adenine dinucleotide (NAD), which you may recall from the previous chapter, is derived from the vitamin niacin. In the following reaction the high-energy phosphate group on C-1 is transferred to ADP to form ATP. The reaction is termed *substrate-level phosphorylation,* to distinguish it from *oxidative phosphorylation* (the formation of ATP by electron flow, shown later). In the following reactions, the remaining phosphate group is prepared for transfer to ADP by isomerization (reaction 8) and dehydration (reaction 9) of the glycerate. These reactions increase the potential energy for transfer of the phosphate group by about fourfold, so that in reaction 10 ATP is easily formed from ADP. By the 10th reaction of this pathway, two molecules of ATP have been consumed and four molecules of ATP have been formed, for a net gain of two ATPs per glucose (or other carbohydrate) molecule.

## Anaerobic Exit of Glycolysis

*Pyruvate,* the last intermediate of the E-M glycolytic pathway, is at a junction point between anaerobic and aerobic metabolism. In anaerobic metabolism there is only a single reaction beyond the E-M pathway, which involves the formation of lactate (Figure 3-13). This reaction was discussed in Chapter 2, but some additional discussion will clarify the abruptness of the pathway, which comes to an end after one reaction. It represents a quick and relatively uncomplicated means by which cells can obtain ATP in the absence of oxygen, though the yield is quite small (two ATPs per glucose molecule). If the cell obtains its ATP from the breakdown of stored glycogen (pathway D, Figure 3-9) it will realize a net gain of three ATPs anaerobically, since no ATP is required to form glucose 6-phosphate from glycogen (as will be explained later). Since anaerobic glycolysis is relatively simple, the pathway can be run at a much faster rate.

Surprisingly, many cells process a relatively large percentage of glucose (or glycogen) via this pathway, including ocular tissues. One reason is that a significant amount of $NAD^+$ must be regenerated from NADH (see Figure 3-13) to be reused in reaction 6 of the E-M pathway (see Figure 3-12). Muscle tissues, in particular, increase their rate of glycolysis with an anaerobic exit, since during strenuous exertion muscles quickly exceed their capacity for aerobic glycolysis. In the eye, corneal epithelia have a decreased amount of available oxygen during contact lens wear and this causes epithelial cells to increase their percentage of anaerobic glycolysis. This was once a major problem in the use of hard contact lenses, since nearly 80% of the available glycogen would be used in just a little more than 8 hours' lens wear compared to soft lenses (Figure 3-14). The resultant metabolic strain on the epithelial cells caused significant swelling of both epithelial and anterior stromal corneal tissues. The increase in total corneal swelling could be as much as 20% of tissue volume (Hamano and Kaufman, 1987).

## Aerobic Exit of Glycolysis
Instead of being converted to lactate at the end of the E-M pathway, pyruvate may diffuse into cellular mitochondria to begin the aerobic phase of

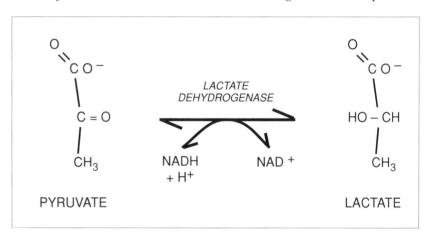

FIGURE 3-13   The single reaction of the anaerobic extension of glycolysis.

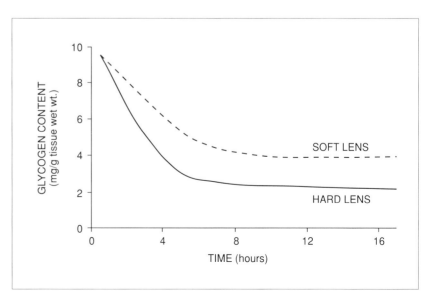

FIGURE 3-14   Decreased concentration of glycogen in the corneal epithelium as a function of contact lens wear.
(Adapted from H. Hamano, et al. The effects of hard and soft contact lenses on rabbit cornea. J Jpn Cl Soc 1972;14:29–37.)

ATP production. In order to understand this process it is helpful to digress to a short explanation of mitochondrial function and anatomy. Cellular mitochondria are organelles that have two principal functions: the manufacture of ATP aerobically and the enzymatic processing of other reactions requiring a separate compartment. Mitochondria exist in various spherical and oblong shapes, but all have a double membrane (Figure 3-15), the inner one of which is impermeable to virtually all molecules and ions. The inner membrane often has a very large surface area represented by infoldings known as *cristae*.

The innermost matrix contains numerous soluble enzymes not found in the cellular cytoplasm. The inner membrane contains a number of insoluble electron-transferring proteins and an enzyme known as *ATP synthase*. Many of the matrix enzymes as well as the inner membrane proteins, including ATP synthase, are essential to aerobic ATP production. The first metabolite to be produced in the aerobic exit of the E-M pathway is acetyl co-enzyme A or CoA (Figure 3-9).

The reaction takes place in the mitochondrial matrix and is shown in simplified form in Figure 3-16. This reaction is the result of the activity of three enzymes and five coenzymes held together in a molecular particle known as the *pyruvate dehydrogenase complex*. Two of the five coenzymes, CoA and $NAD^+$ are given in the diagram. The other three coenzymes are flavin adenine dinucleotide (FAD), thiamine pyrophosphate (TPP), and lipoamide (see Table 2-1).

An important consideration of this complex reaction is the transfer of two electrons from pyruvate to NADH. These electrons (as will be explained) are an early source of ATP synthesis. At this stage, the two-carbon units (i.e., acetyl CoA) that originated from one molecule of glucose (or another source) are now ready to be incorporated into the Krebs cycle. This cyclic pathway, which was discovered by Hans Krebs in 1937, is multifunctional. Its primary purpose in energy production is to supply electrons for the synthesis of ATP. The cycle is diagrammed in Figure 3-17.

There are nine reactions which are all enzyme catalyzed. These reactions occur in the mitochondrial matrix. The important energy-deriving reactions are 4, 5, 6, 7, and 9. In these reactions, electrons are removed either

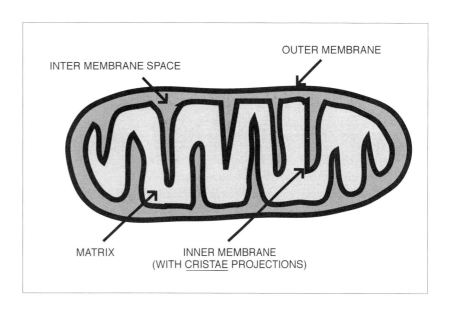

**FIGURE 3-15    Cross-sectional diagram of a typical mitochondrion.**
This subcellular organelle is divided into two compartments (intermembrane space and matrix) by two membranes (outer membrane and inner membrane). The inner membrane has its surface area enlarged by many infoldings (cristae). The shape and number of cristae vary from cell to cell, depending on the metabolic demands of the cell. High energy requiring cells have greater numbers of cristae.

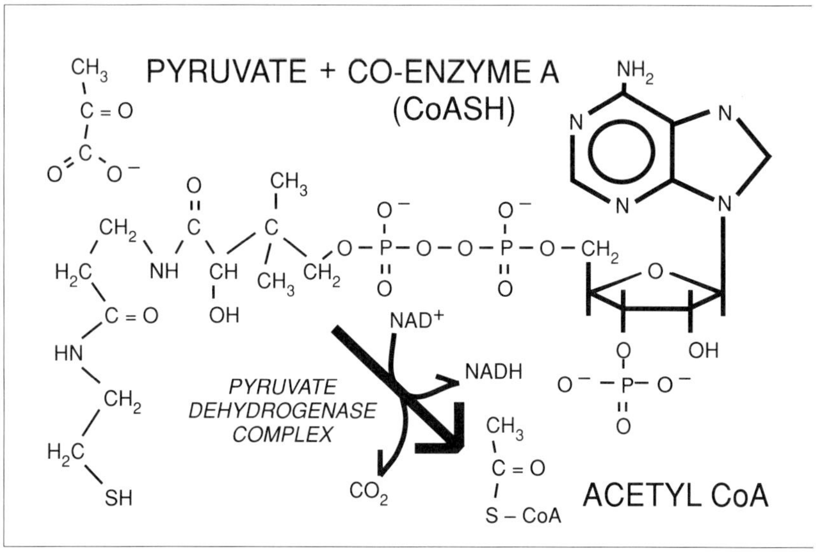

**FIGURE 3-16** Formation of acetyl CoA from pyruvate and CoA.

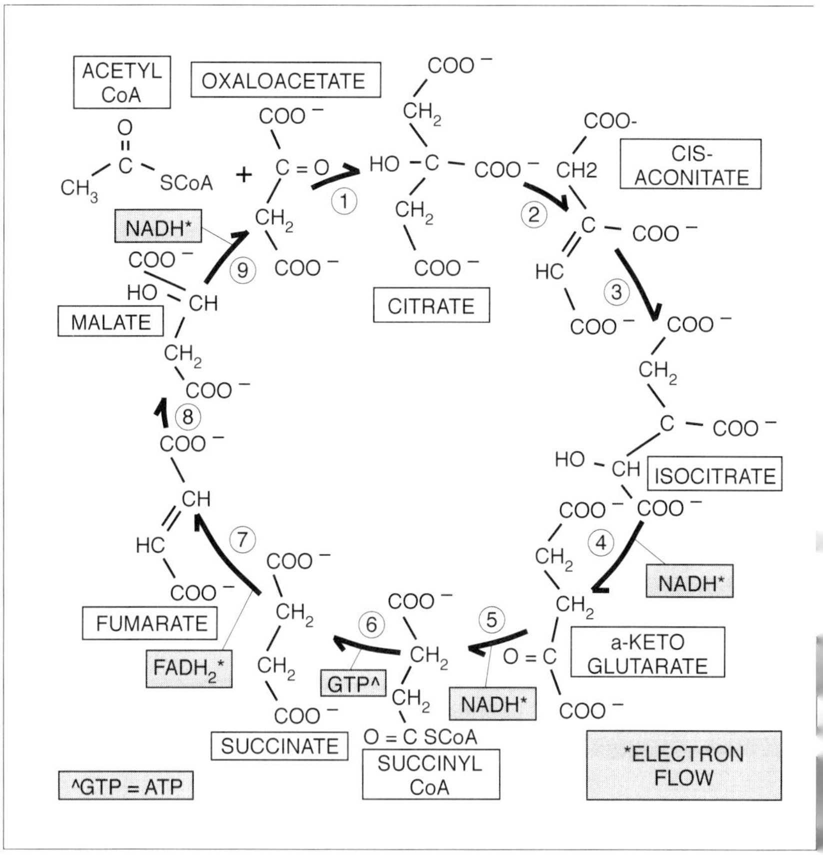

**FIGURE 3-17 The Krebs cycle.**
The cycle begins with acetyl CoA and oxaloacetate (reaction 1) and ends with the formation of oxaloacetate from malate (reaction 9). Electron flow or transport exits the cycle with NADH and FADH$_2$ in reactions 4, 5, 7, and 9. The ATP equivalent GTP is generated in reaction 6. Each reaction is enzyme catalyzed (not shown).

with NADH or FADH$_2$; or a high-energy phosphate is trapped in the released compound guanosine triphosphate (GTP), a high-energy compound similar to ATP. GTP is readily converted to ATP by the reaction

$$GTP + ADP \leftrightarrows GDP + ATP$$

which is also enzyme catalyzed.

The compounds NADH and FADH$_2$, which are coenzymes, diffuse to the inner mitochondrial membrane, where they transfer their electrons to the electron-transferring (redox) proteins located there. When electrons arrive at the inner membrane bound to either NADH or $FADH_2$, they are transported or shuttled between four protein complexes, and ultimately they combine with oxygen and hydrogen to form water (Figure 3-18).

The protein complexes are immobile and are served by coenzyme Q and cytochrome C. Coenzyme Q is a lipophilic quinone with a long hydrocarbon tail of isoprene units (Figure 3-19A). It shuttles electrons between complex I and complex III and also between complex II and complex III. Cytochrome C is a small lipophilic protein of 13 kd (Figure 3-19B) that shuttles electrons between complex III and complex IV. It is NADH that ferries electrons to complex I and $FADH_2$ that carries electrons to complex II. The unique feature of this electron transport is the *electromotive force* generated in the inner mitochondrial membrane as the transport occurs. This force is analogous to electricity flowing through a wire. It generates useful energy equivalent to approximately 53 kcal/mol of oxygen consumed (Stryer, 1988). In more practical terms this is roughly enough energy to heat 1 mL of water to 28°C (about 50°F) for each 1.12 liters of oxygen used.

**FIGURE 3-18** Electron transfer in the inner mitochondrial membrane.

Electrons from NADH are transferred to protein complex I (25 polypeptides) in the inner membrane. Coenzyme Q (Q) transfers electrons from complex I to complex III (10 polypeptides), which also receives electrons from complex II (four polypeptides) via coenzyme Q. Complex II receives electrons from $FADH_2$. From complex III, electrons are transported to complex IV via cytochrome C (C) and from there to form water from oxygen and hydrogen. Each transfer is an oxidation-reduction reaction. In complexes I, III, and IV, hydrogen ions are transported from the matrix to the intermembrane space.

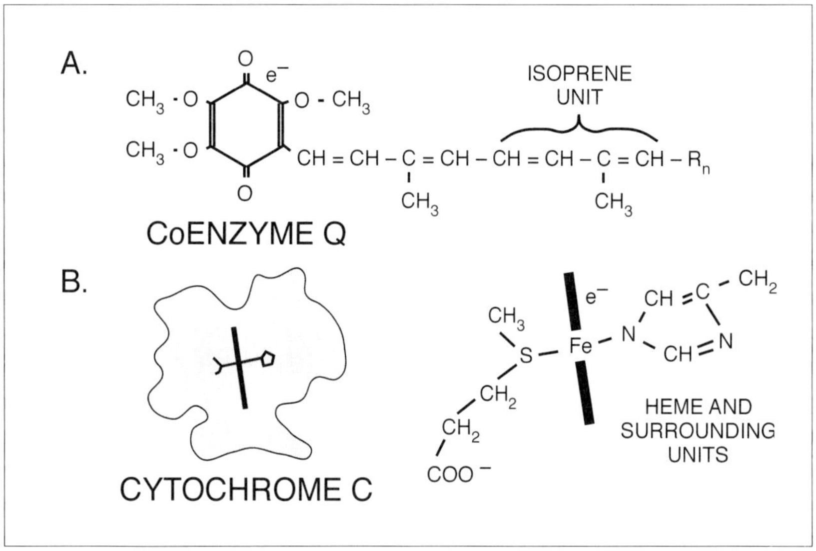

**FIGURE 3-19** Coenzyme Q (*A*) and cytochrome C (*B*) are lipid-soluble molecules in the mitochondrial membrane.

Coenzyme Q is a quinone derivative with a long tail of isoprene units. Electrons are incorporated into the oxygen on the quinone ring. Cytochrome C is a globular protein with a molecular weight of 13 kd. The electron-carrying moiety is a prosthetic (see Chapter 11) heme group with iron at its center. The protein complexes in the membrane (see Figure 3-18) also contain heme groups.

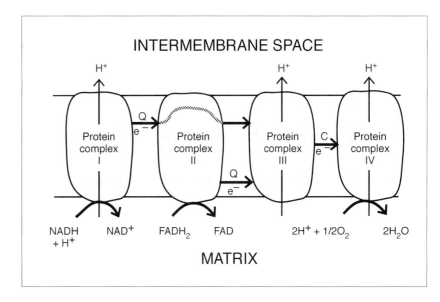

The energy is used to pump hydrogen ions from the mitochondrial matrix to the intermembrane space, creating a relatively acidic environment outside the matrix. The hydrogen ions or protons flow back into the matrix through the pores of a fifth protein complex known as *ATP synthase*. The flow provides the energy to phosphorylate ADP to form ATP. (In fact, the flow simply causes the release of ATP from ATP synthase.) The entire process is shown for NADH-originated electron transport in Figure 3-20. Since the passage of protons through the ATP synthase (complex V) generate one molecule of ATP, the journey of electrons from NADH to water produces three molecules of ATP. This is so since one or more protons are transported through protein complexes I, III, and IV by the passage of each electron pair. The exact number of protons transported outward is presently unknown (Mathews and van Holde, 1990).

In the case of $FADH_2$, only two ATPs are produced, since no proton is transported through protein complex II (see Figure 3-18). The total ATP produced by the aerobic exit of glycolysis is 36 to 38 molecules (Table 3-1).

All sources of ATP have been discussed except the last one, from E-M NADH in the cell cytoplasm. The ATP molecules from this source are obtained by the *glycerol phosphate* and *malate-aspartate* shuttles. In the glycerol phosphate shuttle, dihydroxyacetone phosphate (Figure 3-11), one product of reaction 4, is "borrowed" from the E-M pathway by reaction with NADH (Figure 3-21) to produce glycerol 3-phosphate. This intermediate (bearing

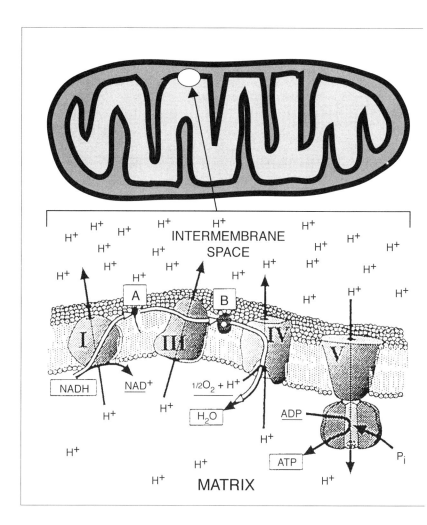

**FIGURE 3-20   A complete overview of oxidative phosphorylation to produce ATP.**

ATP is formed (actually, released) when hydrogens ions (protons) flow through protein complex V (ATP synthase). For this to occur protons are pumped into the intermembrane space as a result of electron flow between protein complexes I, III, and IV using coenzyme Q (A) and cytochrome C (B), starting with NADH and ending with water formation. The electron flow starting with $FADH_2$ and protein complex II is not shown. It should be noted also that protons are not pumped through protein complex II (Figure 3-19), but are pumped subsequently.

two electrons) diffuses to the outer surface of the inner mitochondrial membrane, where it reacts by giving up its two electrons to FAD in the mitochondrial matrix. The glycerol 3-phosphate is converted back to dihydroxyacetone phosphate and "returns" (by diffusion) to the E-M pathway in the cytoplasm. The FAD (as $FADH_2$) is now a source for the production of two additional molecules of ATP. The malate-aspartate shuttle operates by a somewhat similar mechanism, with one important difference, the final electron acceptor molecule in the mitochondrial matrix is NADH rather than $FADH_2$. This difference enables the cell to obtain an additional three molecules of ATP, rather than two molecules. For both shuttles one obtains a net of four or six molecules of ATP, respectively, from a single glucose molecule.

## Glycogen Formation and Degradation

Much of the glucose that enters certain cells is stored as the polysaccharide glycogen. The formation begins at glucose 6-phosphate in the E-M pathway and is relatively direct. Glucose 6-phosphate is isomerized to glucose 1-phosphate. Glucose 1-phosphate reacts with an ATP equivalent known as uridine triphosphate (UTP) to form uridine diphosphoglucose, and this form is added, as glucose, to a growing chain of glycogen by the action of the enzyme *glycogen synthase*. Figure 3-22 outlines the reactions. A branching

**TABLE 3-1   Yield of ATP from Aerobic Glycolysis**

| *Pathway* | *Yield per Molecule of Glucose* |
|---|---|
| Embden-Meyerhof (E-M) | 2 |
| Krebs cycle (as GTP) | 2 |
| Oxidative phosphorylation | |
|    From Krebs cycle NADH | 18 |
|    From Krebs cycle $FADH_2$ | 4 |
|    From CoA formation NADH | 6 |
|    From E-M NADH* | 4–6 |
|            Total | 36–38 |

*Two extra molecules of ATP may be produced by another mechanism to transport E-M pathway NADH into the mitochondria.

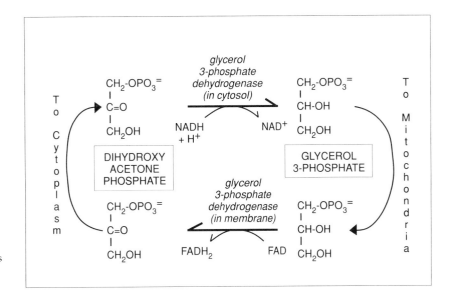

**FIGURE 3-21   The glycerol phosphate shuttle.**
This shuttle exists to transport cytoplasmic NADH electrons to the electron transport protein complexes in the inner mitochondrial membrane.

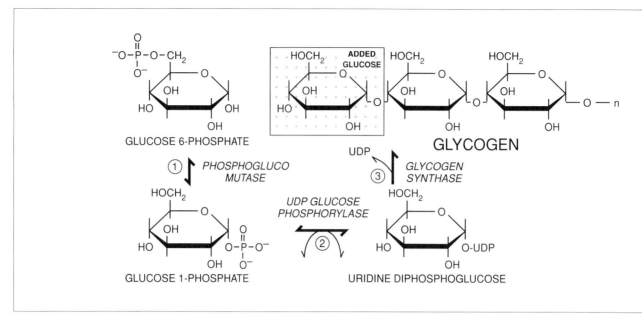

**FIGURE 3-22** The formation of glycogen from glucose 6-phosphate.

Enzymes are named in italics.

enzyme (a transferase) will periodically remove some of the growing terminal chains and bond them onto C-6 of some units (see Figure 3-7).

When glycogen is broken down the process is reversed, but it proceeds by a separate pathway. It is important to have a separate pathway so that the cell can have optimal control of its carbohydrate reserves. Glycogen is broken down, one residue or unit at a time, by the enzyme *glycogen phosphorylase.* Each glucose unit is released as glucose 1-phosphate and then reenters the E-M pathway after the formation of glucose 6-phosphate. Debranching of glycogen occurs from the activity of a glucosidase enzyme. This glucosidase is an allosteric enzyme in which ATP and glucose 6-phosphate maintain it in its T form (see Chapter 2).

The activity of glycogen phosphorylase is also controlled by high levels of ATP and glucose 6-phosphate, which inhibit it. Glycogen synthase and glycogen phosphorylase are reciprocally activated and deactivated by the addition and removal of phosphate groups from each enzyme. When phosphate is added to phosphorylase (low levels of ATP) it is activated while the synthase is inactivated when phosphate is added to its structure. The reverse is true with high levels of ATP for each enzyme (Table 3-2).

**TABLE 3-2   Effects of Phosphate Levels on Enzymatic Glycogen Synthesis and Degradation**

| | | Effects of | |
|---|---|---|---|
| *Enzyme* | *Function* | *High Phosphate* | *Low Phosphate* |
| Glycogen synthase | Adds glucose to glycogen | Inhibits | Activates |
| Glycogen phosphorylase | Removes glucose from glycogen | Activates | Inhibits |

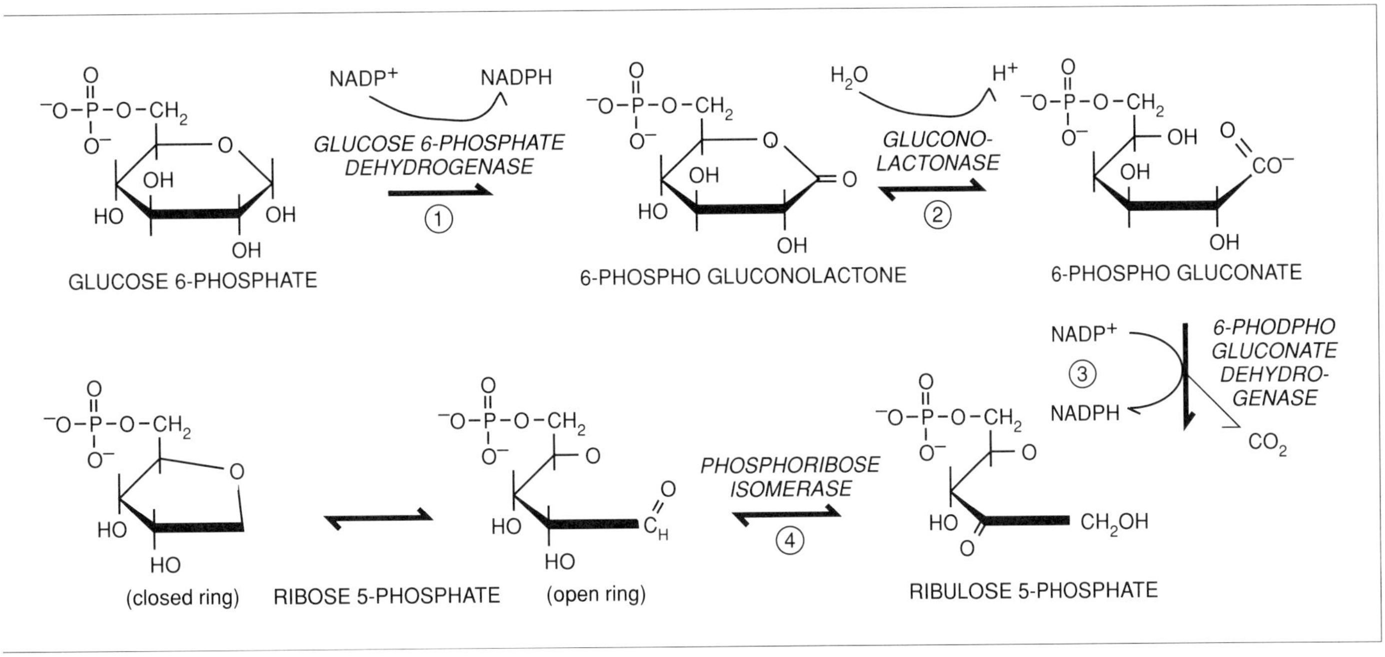

GLUCOSE 6-PHOSPHATE   NADP⁺  NADPH   GLUCOSE 6-PHOSPHATE DEHYDROGENASE (1) → 6-PHOSPHO GLUCONOLACTONE   $H_2O$  $H^+$  GLUCONO-LACTONASE (2) → 6-PHOSPHO GLUCONATE

RIBOSE 5-PHOSPHATE (closed ring) ← (open ring) → PHOSPHORIBOSE ISOMERASE (4) → RIBULOSE 5-PHOSPHATE   NADP⁺ (3) NADPH  6-PHODPHO GLUCONATE DEHYDRO-GENASE  $CO_2$

**FIGURE 3-23  The formation of pentoses from glucose 6-phosphate.**
This is the initial part of the pentose shunt pathway.

## The Pentose Shunt

Another metabolic branch that leads from glucose 6-phosphate is the pentose shunt. This pathway has three principal functions: the generation of pentoses (to be used for nucleic acids and nucleotides such as ATP itself), the production of fatty acids (for membrane synthesis and other functions requiring fatty acids), and cell detoxification by the removal of destructive forms of oxygen (such as hydrogen peroxide). In addition, some metabolic intermediates can be recovered back into the E-M pathway. Here we consider only the first part of the pathway (Figure 3-23).

In reaction 1, electrons are removed from C-1, which forms a carbonyl group. These electrons, which are contained in the coenzyme NADPH (a phosphorylated cousin of NADH), serve two principal functions. One is the reductive (electron-requiring) synthesis of fatty acids. The second is removal of hydrogen peroxide by a linked redox system. In the redox system, electrons from NADPH are used to reduce the peptide glutathione. Glutathione, in turn, reduces hydrogen peroxide to water. The entire linked scheme for reaction 1 is shown below.

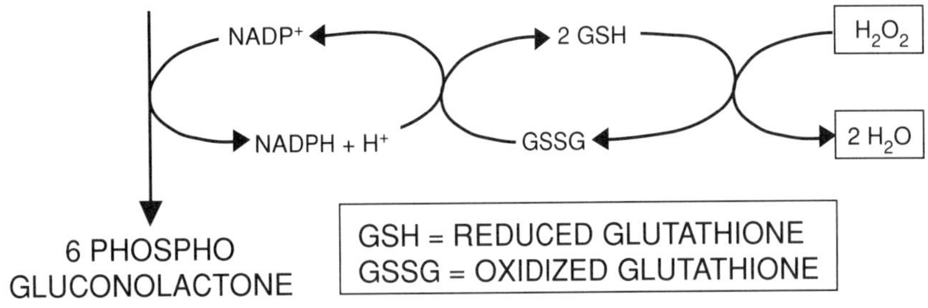

GLUCOSE 6-PHOSPHATE → NADP⁺ / NADPH + H⁺ → 2 GSH / GSSG → $H_2O_2$ / 2 $H_2O$ ; → 6 PHOSPHO GLUCONOLACTONE

GSH = REDUCED GLUTATHIONE
GSSG = OXIDIZED GLUTATHIONE

Each reaction is enzyme catalyzed. The importance of these coupled reactions lies in the fact that cell membranes (containing lipids and proteins) can be destroyed by excessive amounts of hydrogen peroxide and other forms of active oxygen (e.g., superoxide radicals). Such detoxification mechanism are known to be present in ocular tissues (Whikehart, 1978) to prevent tissu destruction. In the second reaction of the pentose shunt the lactone (a internal ester) is hydrolyzed (broken with a water molecule) to produce sugar acid (gluconate). In the third reaction, the acid is oxidized (it lose electrons) and these electrons are again absorbed by $NADP^+$. A molecule $CO_2$ is also lost. The product, ribulose 5-phosphate, is isomerized in reactio 4 to ribose 5-phosphate by transferring the carbonyl group from C-2 to C-so that a closed-ring pentose can be formed. The pentose can then be incorporated into nucleotides and nucleic acids (see Chapter 5). Growing ocula tissues make extensive use of this pathway both for the production of nuclei acids (to synthesize proteins) and lipids (to be incorporated into cellular membranes). An example is the epithelial cells of the cornea.

## Other Aspects of Carbohydrate Metabolism

There are two other aspects of normal carbohydrate metabolism that ar meaningful to some ocular tissues, *gluconeogenesis* and the *Warburg effec* Gluconeogenesis (synthesis of new glucose) proceeds basically as a re versal of the E-M pathway, but it uses four different enzymes not found i the E-M pathway to proceed from lactate to glucose (Figure 3-24). Two o those enzymes are found in the mitochondria. Here again, separate en zymes are employed to maintain independent control of glycolysis (carbo hydrate breakdown) and glucose formation (carbohydrate reformation o

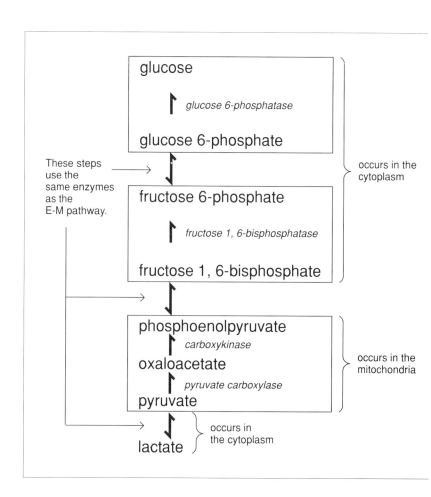

**FIGURE 3-24   Gluconeogenesis.**
This pathway uses some of the enzymes of the E-M pathway. The enzymes unique to the pathway are shown in italics.

gluconeogenesis). Although the liver (and to some extent the kidneys) are the principal sites of this pathway, it is the retina and the brain that are the principal beneficiaries of an adequate level of glucose in the bloodstream.

Gluconeogenesis is especially important to the eye since the photoreceptors have one of the highest demands for a constant supply of glucose and oxygen. The other aspect of carbohydrate formation, the Warburg effect, simply "directs" excess pyruvate to become lactate with a relatively high partial pressure of oxygen. This characteristic of the retina was discussed in Chapter 2, under Lactate Dehydrogenase. One pathway of abnormal carbohydrate metabolism in the eye is the polyol pathway. This was explained in Chapter 2 and will be detailed further in the section of this chapter on Problems of Carbohydrate Transport and Metabolism.

## Comparative Metabolism

The types of carbohydrate metabolism and their relative levels in ocular tissues depend on the roles and associated energy demands of each tissue type. Examples of extreme levels of relative energy demands are found in photoreceptors (highest) and lens fiber cells (lowest). The relative percentages of carbohydrate metabolism in several cell types found in the anterior segment of the eye may be seen in Table 3-3. In the cornea, like most nonocular tissues, there exists a predominance of glucose funneled through the anaerobic exit of glycolysis (E-M pathway). However, it must be kept in mind that the ATP energy derived from aerobic glycolysis does not require as much glucose since aerobic glycolysis produces 36 molecules of ATP per glucose molecule, compared to just two molecules of ATP produced anaerobically.

One may calculate from the data in the table what the total ATP yield would be in each cell type by adding the aerobic and anaerobic ATP produced for every 100 molecules of glucose consumed. Let us consider corneal epithelial cells and keratocytes (which have a similar metabolism):

**TABLE 3-3 Comparative Carbohydrate Metabolism in the Anterior Segment of the Eye**

| Cell Type | Anaerobic Glycolysis (%) | Aerobic Glycolysis (%) | Pentose Shunt (%) | Glycogen Storage | Other (%) |
|---|---|---|---|---|---|
| Cornea* | | | | | |
|   Epithelial | 57 | 8 | 35 | Yes ⎫ | |
|   Stromal | 57 | 8 | 35 | No ⎬ Polyol pathway may be present in diabetes |
|   Endothelial | 70 | 23 | 7 | No ⎭ | |
| Lens† | | | | | |
|   Epithelial | 81 | 4 | 15 | No ⎫ Polyol pathway in diabetes |
|   Fiber‡ | 83 | 2 | 15 | No ⎭ | |
| Ciliary body§ | | | | | |
|   Pigmented ⎫ | 85% of EM‖ | 15% of EM‖ | Present | No | Unknown |
|   Nonpigmented ⎭ | | | | | |

*Data from M. Riley, 1983; and D. Whikehart, 1989.
†Data from J. Kuck, 1970; R. van Heyningen and Linklater, 1975; and Winkler and Riley, 1991. The pentose shunt % is an assumed minimal value for epithelial cells.
‡Values are actually for whole lens; lens fiber cells may have a lower proportion of aerobic glycolysis, especially in the nucleus.
§Data derived from D. Cole, 1970.
‖Percentage of that glucose in the Embden-Meyerhof pathway. The actual percentage in glycolysis is unknown.

Anaerobically      57 glucose molecules (57% of 100 molecules)
$$\begin{array}{r} \times \quad 2 \text{ ATP molecules (produced per glucose molecule)} \\ \hline = 114 \text{ ATP molecules produced} \end{array}$$

Aerobically        8 glucose molecules (8% of 100 molecules)
$$\begin{array}{r} \times \quad 36 \text{ ATP molecules (produced per glucose molecule)} \\ \hline = 288 \text{ ATP molecules produced} \end{array}$$

Combined production  114 + 288 ATP molecules = $\boxed{402 \text{ ATP molecules}}$

The 402 ATP molecules produced per 100 molecules of glucose neglect the possible recovery of some intermediates via the pentose shunt and the fact that some glucose is stored temporarily as glycogen.

The significant percentage of pentose shunt in the corneal epithelial and stromal (keratocyte) cells may be related to the physiological roles of these cells. *Epithelial cells,* which are five to six layers deep in humans, are in constant state of division at their basal layer. There is, therefore, a heavy requirement for protein and lipid synthesis. It may be recalled that two roles of the pentose shunt are for the synthesis of pentoses (to produce nucleic acids) and the generation of the electron bearing coenzyme NADPH (needed to synthesize fatty acids). The nucleic acids are used to synthesize proteins while the fatty acids become the constituents of newly formed cellular membranes. Proteins themselves have many roles in the maintenance and reproduction of cells. *Keratocytes,* although comprising just 5% to 10% of the bulk of the stroma, are responsible for its maintenance and repair. These cells also have a significant need to synthesize proteins like collagen and proteoglycans as well as structural carbohydrates such as glycosaminoglycans. Therefore, these cells must maintain an adequate supply of pentoses to make nucleic acids, which produce the required proteins in turn.

*Corneal endothelial cells,* on the other hand, have an even higher energy demand than the other two corneal cell types. They must maintain the cornea in a relatively equilibrated state of clarity (*deturgescence*). This ocular "sump pump" is thought to be constituted by the activity of the plasma membrane enzyme: Na,K-ATPase (see Chapter 2). This enzyme has a high demand for its substrate: ATP necessitating a higher proportion of the aerobic pathway of glycolysis. In endothelial cells, therefore, one may calculate that the yield of ATP produced per 100 molecules of glucose is equal to 140 molecules (produced anaerobically) and 838 molecules (produced aerobically) for a total amount of 968 molecules of ATP. This amount is about 2.4 times that produced in each of the other cell types of the cornea.

Though there is a constant increase in the production of *lens fiber cells,* the rate of production after birth is very slow. Potassium ions are pumped into and through the lens (anteriorly to posteriorly) by the lens *epithelial cells.* However, the tissues do not have the tendency to imbibe water and swell as does the cornea. Moreover, the lens fiber cells, as they mature, tend to lose their subcellular organelles. Consequently, energy demand is considerably lower in the lens cells than in the cornea. In the lens epithelium, the ATP yield per 100 glucose molecules is 162 (anaerobically) plus 144 (aerobically), or 306 molecules. In the lens fiber cells, the ATP yield per 100 glucose molecules is 166 (anaerobically) plus 72 (aerobically), or 238 in all. In the lens nucleus, it is highly probable that the ATP yield is considerably lower (i.e., approaching 170 molecules of ATP per 100 glucose molecules).

The ATP yield of the ciliary body cannot be accurately calculated since the percentage of glucose sent through the pentose shunt is unknown. It is

**TABLE 3-4  Comparative Carbohydrate Metabolism in the Retina and Brain**

| Cell Type | Anaerobic Glycolysis (%) | Aerobic Glycolysis (%) | Pentose Shunt (%) | Glycogen Storage | Other |
|---|---|---|---|---|---|
| Retina* | | | | | |
|   Photoreceptors and all others | 60 | 25 | 15 | None[†] | Polyol pathway may occur |
| Brain[‡] | | | | | |
|   Whole brain | 17 | 82.7 | <0.3 | Minimal | None |

*Data from Graymore, 1970; and Winkler, 1983.
[†]Except Müller cells.
[‡]Data from Hawkins and Mann, 1983.

perfectly reasonable to assume that the energy requirement is substantial, inasmuch as the cells of this organ generate the intraocular pressure and prepare the aqueous as an ultrafiltrate of blood, just as the kidney prepares urine as an ultrafiltrate of blood.

In the *retina*, the cut or percentage of glucose through aerobic glycolysis is higher than any other part of the eye, in accord with the energy demands of this tissue. This is indicated in Table 3-4 and compared with brain tissue. Nine hundred molecules of ATP are produced aerobically versus 120 molecules of ATP produced anaerobically (total of 1020) per 100 glucose molecules. In the brain the ATP yield is even higher, but the rate of ATP production, that is the number of glucose molecules processed through the pathways in the retina, is higher than that of brain per unit time. This means that the rate of ATP production is actually higher in the retina. This is known from oxygen consumption rates or $QO_2$ values (microliters of oxygen consumed per milligram tissue dry weight per hour; Table 3-5). It is further reflected in blood flow rates through these tissues (Table 3-6).

**TABLE 3-5  Oxygen Consumption Rates ($QO_2$)\* for Ocular and Nonocular Tissues**

| Ocular Tissues | Rate | Nonocular Tissues | Rate |
|---|---|---|---|
| Retina | 31 | Kidney | 21 |
| Cornea | 2 | Cerebral cortex | 12 |
| Lens | 0.5 | Heart | 5 |

*$\mu$L $O_2$/mg tissue dry weight/hour.

**TABLE 3-6  Blood Flow\* Through Various Ocular and Nonocular Tissues**

| Ocular Tissues[†] | Rate | Nonocular Tissues[‡] | Rate |
|---|---|---|---|
| Retina (choroid) | 12 | Heart | 0.6 |
| Ciliary processes | 1.5 | Kidney | 4 |
| Iris | 1 | Brain (gray matter) | 0.5 |

*mL/g tissue/min.
[†]Calculated from Henkind et al., 1979.
[‡]Calculated from Folkow and Neil, 1971.

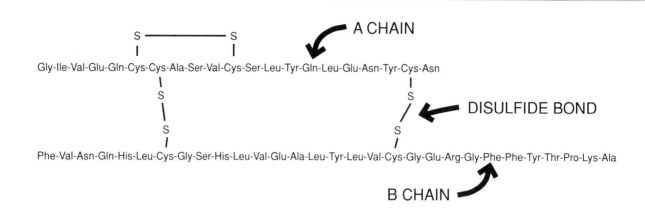

**FIGURE 3-25   Amino acid sequence of insulin.**
Insulin promotes the uptake of glucose into muscle and fat
cells. It also promotes other activities related to cell growth
and metabolism. It is synthesized in the pancreas.

## Problems of Carbohydrate Transport and Metabolism: Diabetes Mellitus and Galactosemia

Glucose and other carbohydrates are taken into cells by facilitated diffusion
and active transport systems. These mechanisms use transport proteins
located on the plasma membranes of the cells. The carbohydrates pass
through membrane proteins to enter the cells, either by themselves (facilitated diffusion) or accompanied by sodium ions (a form of active transport).

Disorders involving the inability to transport glucose into cells fall under
the general disease category known as diabetes mellitus (a name that literally means "sugar in the urine" from the fact that excess glucose is dumped
into the urine from the high amount in the blood). Diabetes is undoubtedly
one of the major disorders affecting humankind. It occurs essentially in two
forms, type I, formerly known as "juvenile-onset diabetes"; and type II,
once called "mature-onset diabetes." Though the mechanisms for each
form vary, both forms involve an inability of glucose to enter certain classes
of cells in the body that are dependent on insulin-activated protein transport systems.

It is important to understand that, in diabetes, although only certain cell
types cannot obtain sufficient glucose, all cell types suffer from the unequal
distribution of glucose: some do not have enough and some are exposed to
excessive (toxic) amounts of glucose. Insulin activates certain glucose-
transporting proteins, since it is a hormone that communicates such activation at the cell surface. It is a polypeptide whose structure is shown in Figure
3-25. (In Chapter 6 other hormones and their activities are discussed.) Insulin, in fact, signals the initiation of many cell functions: glucose and amino
acid uptake, glycolysis, glycogen and lipid synthesis, and synthesis of proteins, deoxyribonucleic acid (DNA), and ribonucleic acid (RNA). One might
say that insulin communicates the continuation of cell nutrition and growth
overall. However, the uptake of glucose remains one of its most important
functions.

In type I diabetes, there is an insufficient amount of circulating insulin
(from the pancreas), probably from damage to the β cells of the pancreas as
a result of either an autoimmune disorder or a viral infection (Mathews and
van Holde, 1990). As a result, high levels of glucose remain in the circulating
blood long after the consumption of a meal. For this reason, type I diabetes

is also known as *insulin-dependent diabetes mellitus* (IDDM). Those cells which depend on insulin become starved for nourishment and other cells not dependent on insulin are exposed to higher than normal cytoplasmic levels of glucose. Cells that are particularly insulin dependent are muscle cells (cardiac, skeletal, and smooth), as well as adipose (fat) cells (McGilvery and Goldstein, 1983), and cells of blood vessel walls (Koschinsky, 1988). Among the cells that are not insulin dependent are red blood cells, bone cells, and lens fiber cells. This is why the enzyme aldose reductase is activated within lens fiber cells in diabetes (Chapter 2).

The insulin-dependent cells alter their metabolism in pathological (abnormal) ways in order to compensate for the lack of glucose. In muscle cells, for example, it is common in the diabetic state to accelerate the breakdown of amino acids (Martin et al., 1985) in order to obtain acetyl CoA (see diagram in Review of Metabolism) as a precursor for ATP. This occurs at the expense of muscle proteins in the body. In fat cells, on the other hand, there is an acceleration of lipid (fat) oxidation (Martin et al., 1985) to produce acetyl CoA for the same purpose—synthesizing ATP. However, in this case, not only are the stores of lipid reduced, but there is also a production of toxic intermediates known as "ketone bodies" (Figure 3-26). Most ketone bodies are sufficiently acidic to lower blood pH to dangerously low levels. This could occur to a point at which the patient might become comatose and, if untreated, could expire. Of course, this represents an extreme case of untreated type I diabetes. Fortunately, only about 10% of the diabetic population has this form and they can usually be managed well with insulin injections.

In type II diabetes, also known as *non–insulin-dependent diabetes mellitus (NIDDM)*, there may be an insufficient number of insulin receptors (so-called down-regulated receptors, Figure 3-27) on the surface (plasma membranes) of insulin-dependent cells or if receptors are present in normal numbers, they may fail to promote sufficient glucose uptake (Mathews and van Holde, 1990; Martin et al., 1985). An insulin molecule binds to the receptor exteriorly and causes activation of the enzyme tyrosine kinase on the portion of the receptor located in the cell cytoplasm. The details of the remaining events are still unsettled, but the kinase adds phosphate groups to intermediate proteins (mediators) that bring about a variety of events associated with cell nutrition and growth. One event is the signalling of

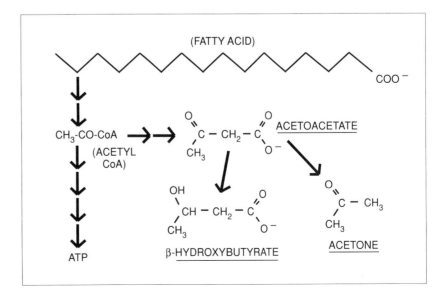

**FIGURE 3-26 The formation of ketone bodies.**
Acetoacetate, acetone, and β-hydroxybutyrate are formed from acetyl CoA as a result of the excessive catabolism of fatty acids. Multiple arrows indicate several enzyme-catalyzed steps.

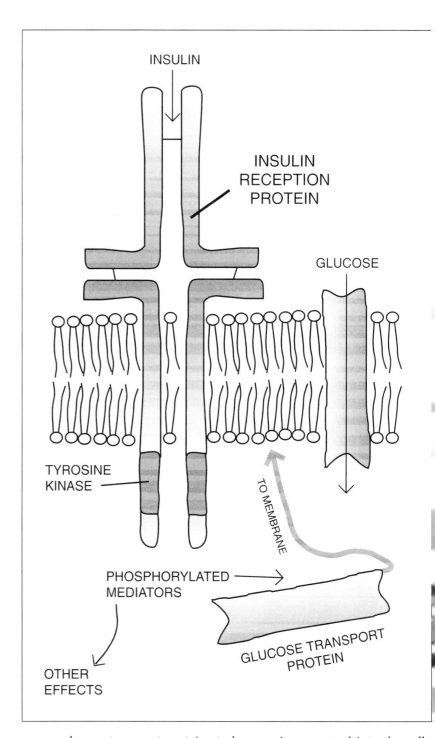

INSULIN

INSULIN RECEPTION PROTEIN

GLUCOSE

TYROSINE KINASE

TO MEMBRANE

PHOSPHORYLATED MEDIATORS

GLUCOSE TRANSPORT PROTEIN

OTHER EFFECTS

**FIGURE 3-27   Insulin receptor protein at a cell plasma membrane.**
The receptor protein consists of four polypeptides held together by disulfide bonds (*thin lines*). It incorporates tyrosine kinase enzymes on the cytoplasmic side of the membrane. This enzyme is activated when insulin binds to the receptor and causes phosphorylation of other cytoplasmic proteins as an initiation of its "message." One message is to move glucose transport proteins to the cell surface.

reserve glucose transport proteins to become incorporated into the cell membrane (surface) so they can increase the amount of glucose that is brought into the cell. This particular event has been documented to occur in fat cells. Type II diabetes is considerably less severe than type I. Usually, a controlled diet coupled with exercise is sufficient to manage it.

Another effect of diabetes that can occur with either form is the binding of glucose to proteins (glycation). In higher glucose concentrations this occurs by what is known as the "Amadori rearrangement" (Figure 3-28). The final bond, a ketimine, is very stable. These protein-carbohydrate conjugates seem to occur in a number of extracellular proteins as well as the intracellular proteins of non–insulin-dependent cells (Cohen, 1986). Among the

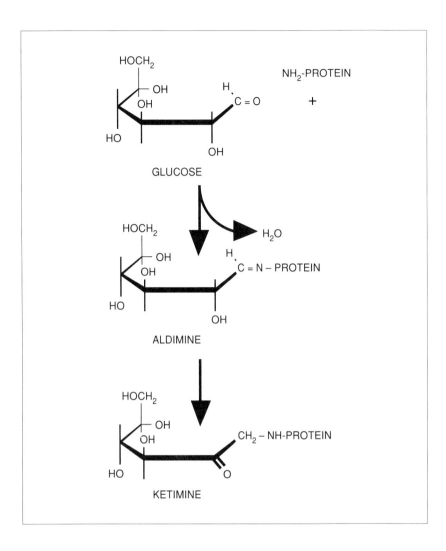

HOCH₂

OH
OH

HO

H
C = O

OH

GLUCOSE

NH₂-PROTEIN

+

H₂O

HOCH₂

OH
OH

HO

H
C = N – PROTEIN

OH

ALDIMINE

HOCH₂

OH
OH

HO

CH₂ – NH-PROTEIN

O

KETIMINE

**FIGURE 3-28   Glycation reaction.**
An example is the binding of glucose to protein with a
subsequent Amadori rearrangement to form a permanent
ketimine.

proteins known to be bound are: collagen, lens crystallins, and enzymes such as Na,K-ATPase and hemoglobin (the oxygen-carrying protein). Some believe this binding explains effects such as leaky capillary filtration barriers (the result of bound collagen), initiation of cataract formation (bound crystallins), corneal swelling (bound Na,K-ATPase), and tissue hypoxia (bound hemoglobin). It has also been proposed (Morita et al., 1985) that glucose in high concentrations may be responsible for DNA damage.

Ocular effects from diabetes occur to the lens, the retina, and the cornea. In the lens, diabetes can cause cataract formation. The strongest evidence for a biochemical mechanism can be related to the polyol pathway (see Chapter 2, Aldose Reductase). This pathway (Figure 3-29) was discovered in the lens in 1963 (Kinoshita et al.). Although it can occur in other tissues, it seems to be most active in the lens. Sorbitol is generated in the first reaction. Recall that sorbitol causes damage to lens fiber cells by increasing osmotic pressure within the cells until they burst. This occurs since sorbitol is not able to leave the cell easily and, although the second enzyme removes sorbitol by converting it to fructose, the rate of conversion is too low to prevent eventual damage. This may be seen from data obtained by Varma et al. (1977) in the lens of a South American rodent, the degu (Table 3-7). It can be readily seen that the level of sorbitol is more than twice that of fructose and about 12 times that of glucose.

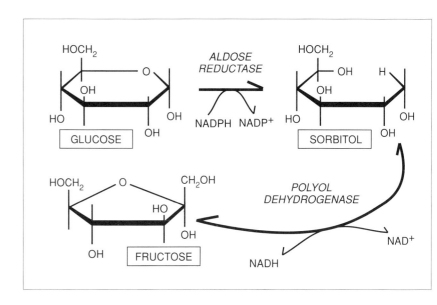

**FIGURE 3-29  The polyol pathway.**
When the substrate is galactose (rather than glucose, as shown) the polyol product galactitol serves as a very poor substrate for polyol dehydrogenase.

A second carbohydrate that uses the polyol pathway when present in high concentrations is galactose. Such high concentrations occur in galactosemia, a disease resulting from the hereditary deficiency of any one of three enzymes involved in converting galactose to glucose 6-phosphate for use in the E-M pathway. The three enzymes are uridyl transferase, galactokinase, and 4-epimerase (Figure 3-30). An important difference in the metabolism of galactose to galactitol by aldose reductase (see Figure 3-29) is that galactitol is a very poor substrate for the second enzyme in the polyol pathway. As a result of this relative inactivity, galactitol is deposited in the lens more rapidly than sorbitol and cataract development proceeds faster. Usually, galactosemia is diagnosed in infants, and if it is found in time cataract formation can be prevented by withholding milk and milk products containing lactose.

In the retina, diabetes can devastate the retinal blood vessels, which are necessary to nourish retinal neurons and photoreceptors. This action is similar to what diabetes does to blood vessels in other parts of the body (e.g., kidneys, brain and limbs). In the retina, this condition is known as *diabetic retinopathy*. It may be the result of several biochemical mechanisms already discussed (Figure 3-31): activation of aldose reductase to destroy pericytes, binding of glucose to basement membrane collagen resulting in thickened fibers, and alteration (damage) of endothelial and pericyte DNA by glucose to produce modified basement membranes (Apple et al., 1988). The loss of pericytes affects vessel integrity, and possibly flow regulation. The thickening of basement membranes alters membrane permeability and leads to

**TABLE 3-7  Carbohydrate Concentrations Found in the Lens of South American Degus*†**

| | Concentration (μmoles/g tissue wet weight) | |
|---|---|---|
| *Glucose* | *Sorbitol* | *Fructose* |
| 1.7 | 18.7 | 8.4 |

*The β-cells in the pancreas were destroyed with streptozotocin.
†Data from Varma et al., 1977.

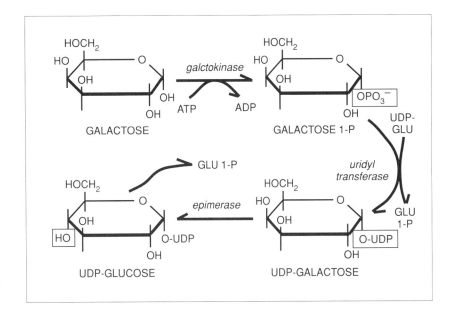

**FIGURE 3-30 The incorporation of galactose into the E-M pathway.**
Several reactions are involved. Glucose 1-phosphate is finally converted to glucose 6-phosphate by phosphoglucomutase (not shown). Enzyme deficiencies in this incorporation pathway (particularly uridyl transferase) cause galactosemia.

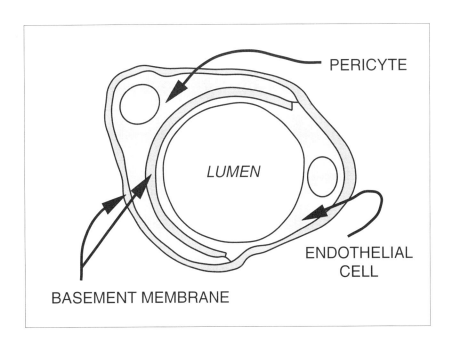

**FIGURE 3-31 Cross-section of a blood vessel typical of those found in capillary beds from the central retinal artery.**
(Adapted from Frank RN et al. Pericyte coverage of capillaries. *Invest Ophthalmol Vis Sci* 1990;31:999–1007.)

occlusion of the lumen. Hemorrhages and retinal detachment follow. The terminal result of these events is loss of vision, in part or all of the retina.

In the cornea, three kinds of tissue damage occur, probably as a result of glucose binding to proteins or from defective protein synthesis resulting from DNA damage. These effects are: nerve degeneration, defective attachment of the epithelium to its underlying stroma, and swelling of the stroma (Figures 1-27, 3-32). The nerves degenerate as a result of irregularities in corneal nerve Schwann cells (basal lamina), as reported by Ishida et al., 1984. This is a protein alteration. In about 50% of diabetic patients, the epithelial layer loses its ability to anchor to the anterior stroma (Kenyon, et al., 1979). This is an alteration of collagen. The stroma swells due to a decrease in the activity of Na,K-ATPase in the endothelium (Herse, 1990). The loss of corneal nerves decreases sensitivity to bacterial infections and can lead to ulceration, while defective anchoring fibrils for the epithelium impairs wound healing

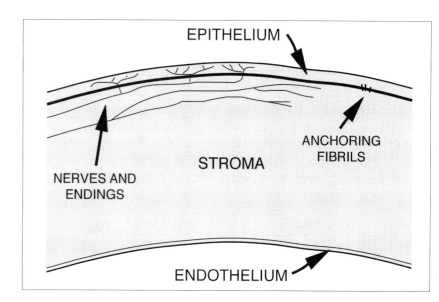

**FIGURE 3-32    Cross-section of the cornea showing the partial distribution of nerves, anchoring fibrils of the epithelium and endothelium.**
These features of the cornea are affected in diabetes.

and promotes erosions of the epithelium (Benson et al., 1988). Stromal swelling can affect the ability to wear contact lenses. The swelling becomes particularly marked in individuals who have diabetic retinopathy.

## Glycosaminoglycans and Oligosaccharides

Long polymers of carbohydrates typically have structural and other supportive tasks in all bodily tissues, including those of the eye. These polymers are found mostly in the extracellular matrix, which is a complex of predominately acellular tissue that shapes and maintains the form of multicellular organisms. In addition, these polymers are involved in cushioning, lubricating, and attaching the matrix to various kinds of cells. In the latter role, they act as a type of biological glue. *Glycosaminoglycans* (described in the next paragraph) have important roles in the eye. For example, as part of the vitreous they help support the retina in its concave configuration and prevent detachment of the retinal neurons from the photoreceptors. At the same time they are involved in absorbing mechanical blows to the eye, and even in cushioning the force of ocular saccades (abrupt shifts in fixation from one point to another, as occurs in reading). While doing this, these vitreous polymers must also allow unhindered passage of light from the lens to the retina.

The term applied to long carbohydrate polymers in the extracellular matrix, glycosaminoglycan (GAG) denotes a repeating unit of a sugar and an aminosugar. Formerly, GAGs were called mucopolysaccharides (MPS), since they are abundant in mucous tissues and were first observed there. Most GAGs occur linked to core proteins, and the entire assembly is known as a *proteoglycan*. Proteoglycans and GAGs are often associated with collagen in extracellular matrices. The common GAG structural units that are found in ocular tissues are shown in Figures 3-33 and 3-34.

Though these structures may seem complex, inspection reveals that they are simple derivatives of carbohydrates. *Glucuronic acid* (also known as glucuronate) is glucose with C-6 converted to a carboxylic acid, whereas *N*-acetylated glucose and galactosamines are glucose and galactose to which nitrogens have been added onto C-2 and the nitrogens (in turn) have had

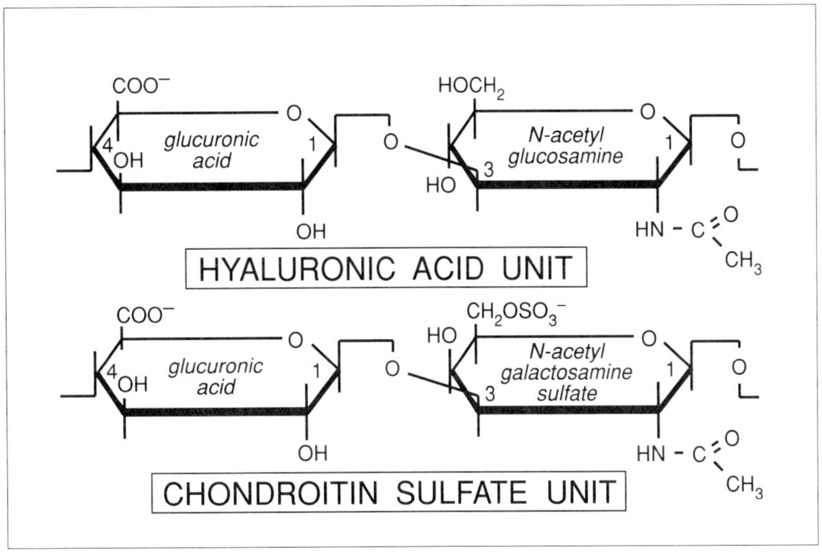

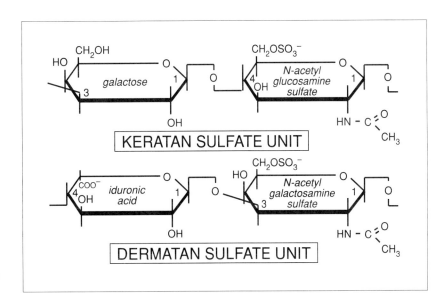

**FIGURE 3-33  Repeating units of the GAGs hyaluronic acid and chondroitin sulfate.**
The negative charges of glucuronic acid and N-acetyl galactosamine sulfate give water imbibing qualities to these GAGs.

**FIGURE 3-34  Repeating units of the GAGs keratan sulfate and dermatan sulfate.**
Iduronic acid is an isomer of glucuronic acid. Sulfate groups can vary in amount and be added to C-4 also.

acetyl (acetate) groups added to them. Iduronic acid is an isomer of glucuronic acid (the acidic group is attached downward in the figure). The individual *members* of each unit are linked (β1→3), whereas *units* are linked (β1→4) except for keratan sulfate, where the order is reversed. Sulfation (the addition of sulfate groups) to the right-hand unit adds considerable acidity and charge density to the entire unit. The sulfate groups can vary in number. The negative charge density is an important characteristic of GAGs, and it explains why the corneal stroma would tend to swell, in the absence of an active deturgescing enzyme, from the high osmotic pressure there.

Figure 3-35 shows the appearance of a segment of hyaluronic acid and its structural participation as a gellike substance interposed between the collagen fibrils of the secondary vitreous of the eye (compare Figure 1-25). Hyaluronic acid is a GAG that is not linked to a core protein; however, new evidence indicates the hyaluronate may be bound to a globular protein (Ren et al., 1991). In the corneal stroma two types of GAGs are found that are linked to core proteins: keratan sulfate and dermatan sulfate. Until recently the core proteins themselves have been difficult to isolate and describe. Jost

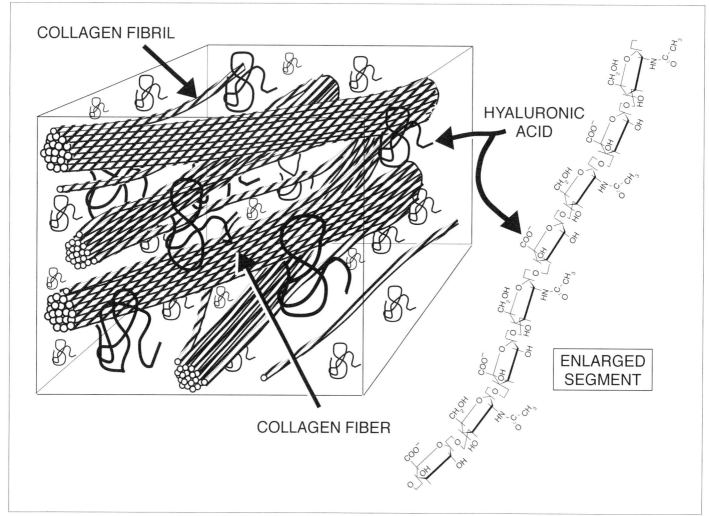

**FIGURE 3-35   Cuboidal section of the vitreous showing GAG and collagen components.**
The hyaluronic acid (HA) molecules position themselves between the collagen fibrils, somewhat like packing material that is used to cushion the contents of a package. An enlarged segment of HA is shown to the right of the figure.

et al. (1991) have described three proteins that bind to keratan sulfate, one of which is called *lumican* (Figure 3-36). A core protein that binds to dermatan sulfate has been called *decorin,* and is present in cornea (Fisher et al., 1989). The exact form of these proteins is unknown, but the core proteins of the proteoglycans in the cornea are thought to bind to only one, two, or three GAGs. These proteoglycans function as spacer molecules between the colalgen fibers of the stromal lamellae (Hascall and Hascall, 1981). This characteristic is important for maintaining *corneal clarity,* since the regular distance array causes the mutual destructive interference of light and prevents scatter or cloudiness (Maurice, 1975).

In certain diseases (e.g., dystrophies) in which the corneal endothelial pump (i.e., Na,K-ATPase) is affected (McCartney et al., 1989), water enters the space where the proteoglycans are located and sufficiently increases the distance between collagen fibers so that the corneal stroma may become cloudy as a result of scattered light. Midura et al. (1990) have also demonstrated that there is abnormal proteoglycan synthesis in some of these dystrophies, which may also contribute to the cloudiness.

Much less common are a group of diseases known as *mucopolysaccharidoses,* a name applied when the term mucopolysaccharide (MPS) was used rather than GAG. These diseases result from a deficiency of one of several enzymes that normally degrade (catabolize) GAGs (Grayson, 1979). As a

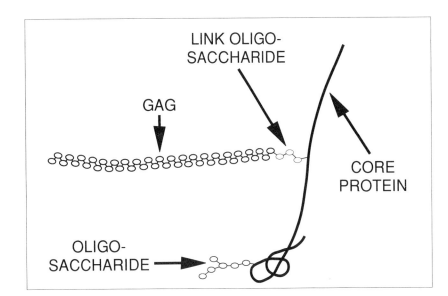

**FIGURE 3-36 A proteoglycan typical of those found in the cornea.**
One to three GAGs are linked to their core protein (e.g., lumican) by an oligosaccharide. Another oligosaccharide (below the GAG) is not linked to any GAG. (Adapted from Hassell, J. et al. Proteoglycan core protein families. *Ann Rev Biochem* 1986;55:539–567.)

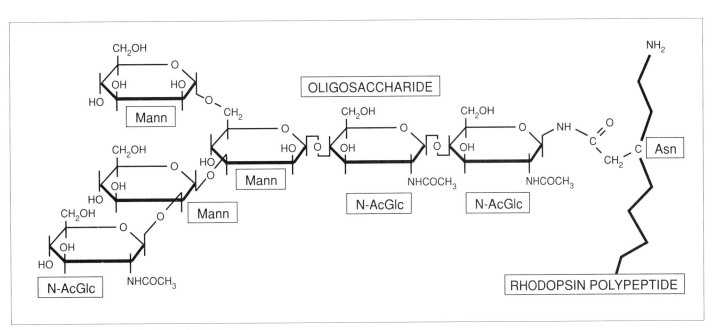

**FIGURE 3-37 An oligosaccharide typically found on rhodopsin molecules.**
The oligosaccharide is bound to asparagine (Asn) by an amide bond. N-AcGLc = N-acetyl glucosamine. Mann = mannose.

result of the deficiency, partially degraded GAGs deposit in bodily tissues. In the cornea this causes opacification or cloudiness and in the retina, retinal degeneration and optic atrophy. The effects vary with the enzyme defect. All MPS diseases are inherited. One example is Hurler's syndrome, a disease that not only affects the eyes, but also causes mental retardation, skeletal deformaties, and cardiac deficiency.

Short lengths of carbohydrates which occur bound to proteins (and lipids) are known as *oligosaccharides* (see Chapter 1). For example, Table 1-5 lists mannose and *N*-acetylglucosamine as the oligosaccharide components of rhodopsin. One of the three variants of the sequence of these oligosaccharides in rhodopsin is shown in Figure 3-37. The purposes of attaching oligosaccharides to proteins are only partially understood. In the case of rhodopsin, the hydrophilic sugars prevent the molecule from flip-flopping in the membrane disc, a process which would impair visual transduction. Short oligosaccharides are also used to couple core proteins to GAGs.

## Summary

Carbohydrates are polyhydroxy compounds containing aldehydes, ketones, and other functional groups. In solution they are capable of forming closed-ring structures, and most contain at least one reactive carbon (C-1) when it is free. These compounds may form short- or long-chain polymers. Ocular tissues use carbohydrates in monosaccharide form as sources of cellular ATP (a high-energy compound that drives many reactions in cells). The glycolytic reactions that are involved can occur in the presence and absence of oxygen, though some oxygen is always required for cell survival. Ocular cells use varying proportions of aerobic and anaerobic metabolism in glycolysis to achieve their particular energy demands. Photoreceptors require the highest levels of ATP, whereas lens fiber cells the least. Glycogen is a long-branched polymer of glucose that exists as a cellular storage form of glucose. The metabolic pathway known as the pentose shunt is useful in the production of pentoses (for nucleic acids) and lipids (for cell membranes). It also is coupled to reactions that detoxify cells from intracellular hydrogen peroxide. When carbohydrates are unable to enter insulin-dependent cells of the body, the body suffers in a diabetic state. In the diabetic eye, the retina can develop degenerative blood vessels with a loss in vision. The same condition can cause cataract formation in the lens. Furthermore, corneal epithelial cells can fail to reattach to their basement membrane, while the whole cornea may swell. These conditions result from either a lack of circulating insulin or from deficient insulin receptors on cell surfaces. Some carbohydrate derivatives form tissue structures and occur in the extracellular matrix. These derivatives are polymers and are classified as glycosaminoglycans (GAGs). Many GAGs combine with core proteins to form proteoglycans. In the eye these polymers are found in the vitreous, cornea, lens capsule, sclera, and blood vessels.

## References

Apple DJ, Pfeffer BR, McFarland ST, Irenberg RA, and Newman DA. Diabetes and eye disease: histopathologic correlations. *In: Diabetes and Its Ocular Complications.* Philadelphia: WB Saunders, 1988;179–189.

Benson WE, Brown GC, and Tasman W. *In Diabetes and Its Ocular Complications.* Philadelphia: WB Saunders, 1988;110.

Bridger WA, and Henderson JF. *Cell ATP.* New York: John Wiley and Sons, 1983;14–15.

Caraway WT, and Watts NB. Carbohydrates. *In* Tietz WW (ed). *Textbook of Clinical Chemistry.* Philadelphia: WB Saunders, 1986;793-794.

Cohen MP. *Diabetes and Protein Glycosylation.* New York: Springer-Verlag, 1986;5–16, 19, 67–94.

Cole, DF. Aqueous and ciliary body. *In:* Graymore CN (ed). *Biochemistry of the Eye.* London: Academic Press, 1970;105–181.

Fisher LW, Termine JD, and Young MF. Deduced protein sequence of bone small proteoglycan I (biglycan) shows homology with proteoglycan II (decorin) and several non-connective proteins in a variety of species. *J Biol Chem* 1989;264:2471–4576.

Folkow B, and Neil E. *Circulation.* New York: Oxford University Press, 1971.

Graymore CN. Biochemistry of the retina. *In:* Graymore CN (ed). *Biochemistry of the Eye.* London: Academic Press, 1970;645–735.

Grayson M. *Diseases of the Cornea.* St. Louis: CV Mosby, 1979;396–404

Hamano H, and Kaufman HE. *The Physiology of the Cornea and Contact Lens Application.* New York: Churchill Livingstone, 1987;16–20.

Hascall VC, and Hascall GK. Proteoglycans. *In: Cell Biology of the Extracellular Matrix.* New York: Plenum, 1981;39–63.

Hawkins RA, and Mann AM. Intermediary metabolism of carbohydrates and other fuels. *In* Lajtha A (ed.). *Handbook of Neurochemistry,* 2nd ed, vol 3. New York: Plenum, 1983; 259–294.

Henkind P, Hausen RI, and Szalay J. Ocular circulation. *In* Records RE (ed). *Physiology of the Human Eye and Visual System.* Hagerstown, MD: Harper & Row, 1979; 98–155.

Herse P. Corneal hydration control in normal and alloxan-induced diabetic rabbits. *Invest Ophthalmol Vis Sci* 1990;31:2205–2213.

Ishida N, Rao GN, del Cerro M, and Aquabella V. Corneal nerve alterations in diabetes mellitus. *Arch Ophthalmol* 1984;102:1380–1384.

Jost CJ, Funderburgh Jl, Mann M, Hassell JR, and Conrad GW. Cell free translation and characterization of corneal keratan sulfate proteoglycan core proteins. *J Biol Chem* 1991;266:13336–13341.

Kenyon K, Wafai Z, Michels R, Conway B, and Tolentino F. Corneal basement membrane abnormality in diabetes mellitus. *Invest Ophthalmol Vis Sci* 1979;17(Suppl):245.

Kinoshita J, Futterman S, Satoh K, and Merola LO. Factors affecting the formation of sugar alcohols in the ocular lens. *Biochem Biophys Acta* 1963;74:350.

Koschinsky T. Effect of insulin on the blood vessel wall. *In:* Weber B (ed). *Pediatric and Adolescent Endocrinology.* Basel: Karger, 1988;17:69–74.

Kuck JFR. Chemical constituents of the lens. *In:* Graymore CN (ed). *Biochemistry of the Eye.* London: Academic Press, 1970;183-260.

Martin DW, Mayes PA, Rodwell VW, and Granner DK. *Harper's Review of Biochemistry,* 20th ed. Los Altos, CA: Lange Medical, 1985;488,601.

Mathews CK, and van Holde KE. *Biochemistry.* Redwood City, CA: Benjamin/Cummings, 1990;527, 786–790.

Maurice DM. The structure and transparency of the cornea. *J Physiol* 1975;136:263-286.

McCartney MD, Wood TO, and McLaughlin BJ. ATPase pump site density in human dysfunctional corneal endothelium. *Invest Ophthalmol Vis Sci* 1989;28:1955–1962.

McGilvery RW, and Goldstein GW. *Biochemistry, A Functional Approach.* Philadelphia: WB Saunders, 1983;461, 739.

Midura RJ, Hascall VC, MacCallam DK, et al. Proteoglycan biosynthesis by human corneas from patients with types 1 and 2 macular dystrophy. *J Biol Chem* 1990;265:15947–15955.

Morita J, Ueda K, Nanjo S, and Komano T. Sequence specific damage of DNA by reducing sugars. *Nucleic Acids Res* 1985;13:449–458.

Ren ZX, Brewton RG, and Mayne R. An analysis by rotary shadowing of the structure of the mammalian vitreous humor and zonular apparatus. *J Struct Biol* 1991;106:57–63.

Riley MV. Corneal endothelial transport. *In:* McDevitt DS (ed). *Cell Biology of the Eye.* New York: Academic Press, 1982;53–95.

Roehrig KL. *Carbohydrate Biochemistry and Metabolism.* Westport, CT: AVI, 1984;3.

Stryer L. Biochemistry. New York: WH Freeman, 1988;359–361, 401, 450.

van Heyningen R, and Linklater J. The metabolism of the bovine lens in air and nitrogen. *Exp Eye Res* 1975;20:393–396.

Varma SD, Mizuno A, and Kinoshita JH. Diabetic cataracts and flavenoids. *Science* 1977;195:205–206.

Whikehart DR. Glutathione peroxidase activity in the bovine corneal endothelium. A comparison with its activity in the corneal epithelium and whole lens. Ophthalmic Res 1978;10:187–193.

Whikehart DR. Irrigating solutions. *In:* Bartlett JD, and Jaanus SD (eds). *Clinical Ocular Pharmacology*, 2nd ed. Boston: Butterworth, 1989;285–299.

Winkler BS. The intermediary metabolism of the retina: biochemical and functional aspects. *In:* Anderson RE (ed). *Biochemistry of the Eye.* San Francisco: American Academy of Ophthalmology, 1983;227–242.

Winkler BS, and Riley MV. Relative contributions of epithelial cells and fibers to rabbit lens ATP content and glycolysis. *Invest Ophthalmol Vis Science* 1991;32:2593-2598.

# Chapter 4

# Lipids

## Review of Lipids

The terms "lipids" and "fats" have been used interchangeably to refer to groups of compounds that are water insoluble but soluble in nonpolar solvents such as benzene, chloroform, and hexane. Strictly speaking, however, the term "fat" refers to lipid esters of fatty acids and glycerol. Such substances are called *hydrophobic* (literally, having an aversion to water). When present in an aqueous or polar environment, lipids associate together. This may be seen, for example, with droplets of oil in a puddle of water. It turns out, however, that most lipids are also partially polar or hydrophilic (literally, water-loving) at one end or region of their structure. *The dual property of hydrophobicity, the dominant characteristic, and hydrophilicity, the minor characteristic, is called an amphipathic property. These characteristics make lipids very useful in cell membranes, where many lipids are found.*

There are several ways to classify lipids, and, in fact, some may be included in more than one class. The most important lipid classes are fatty acids, triacylglycerols, phospholipids, isoprenoids, esters, eicosanoids, and glycolipids (see Figures 4-1, 4-3, 4-4, 4-6 through 4-9).

## Fatty Acids

*Fatty acids consist of varying chain lengths* (about 3 to 30 carbons) of hydrocarbons, the hydrophobic portion, with a carboxylic acid group at one end of the chain, the hydrophilic portion. The characteristics of each fatty acid are determined by its chain length (longer chains are more hydrophobic but have higher melting points) and the degree of unsaturation (i.e., the number of double bonds). The more double bonds present in a fatty acid, the lower its melting point and the greater the degree of fluidity it imparts to a cell membrane.

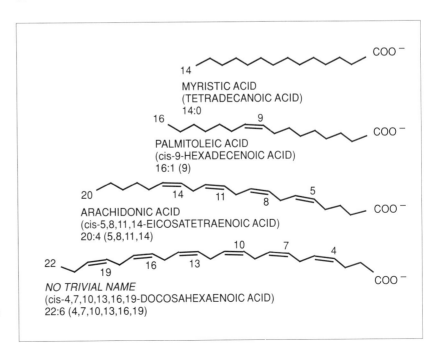

**FIGURE 4-1  Four examples of fatty acids.**
For each acid the trivial name is given first, followed by the IUPAC name. Beneath that is the abbreviation for the IUPAC name. The first number gives the number of carbons. The number after the colon gives the number of double bonds. The number in parentheses designates the carbon number, closest to the carboxylate (COO⁻) group, which shares the double bond. An alternate system (see Figure 4-15) designates the carbon number, starting from the non-carboxylate group (omega number) for the double bond position.

Figure 4-1 shows four examples of fatty acids found in animals and humans. For each example the name given first is the *trivial,* or nonsystematic, *name.* In fact, there is nothing trivial about these "trivial" names. They have been in prevalent use for many generations. The second name is a *systematic name* assigned by the International Union of Pure and Applied Chemistry (IUPAC system). The third name, or abbreviation, is a shorthand version of the systematic name. The figure shows an example of a saturated fatty acid (myristic) and fatty acids with, respectively, one double bond (palmitoleic), four double bonds (arachidonic), and six double bonds (docosahexaenoic). The last fatty acid is present in significant quantities in membranes of photoreceptors of the retina. Some important fatty acids are included in Table 4-1.

The carbon length and degree of unsaturation are important determinants in establishing the melting point and fluidity of biological membranes (Figure 4-2). Though increasing the carbon length of fatty acids can thicken a membrane (and raise its melting point), the inclusion of several double bonds lowers the melting point sufficiently to keep the membrane fluid (or flexible). Fluidity is conferred by the existence of kinks or twists in the fatty acids at each double bond. In this way the membrane is rendered less compact and the fatty acids are free to slide by one another.

## Triacylglycerols

Triacylglycerols (formerly, triglycerides) are fats that represent a storage form of fatty acids. One molecule consists of three fatty acids covalently bonded to a glycerol molecule with ester bonds (Figure 4-3). The fatty acids on each glycerol molecule are often mixed types of chain length and saturation so that the lipid may exist in liquid form. Most triacylglycerols are kept in fat cells and represent a large depot of stored energy (as well as a source of insulation) for the organism. In Chapter 3, it was stated that lipids may be broken down to form acetyl CoA to obtain ATP. This process can occur without excessive ketone body production (as it does in diabetes), so that an individual may be sustained when food is not consumed for longer than normal periods of time. An individual who weighs approximately 155 lb (i.e., the 70-kg individual often quoted in nutrition tables of the National Research Council, 1980) can store 100,000 kcal of energy in the form of

**TABLE 4-1  Partial List of Fatty Acids in Ocular and Nonocular Tissues**

| Trivial Name | IUPAC Name | Abbreviation |
|---|---|---|
| Myristic acid | Tetradecanoic acid | 14:0 |
| Palmitic acid | Hexadecanoic acid | 16:0 |
| Stearic acid | Octadecanoic acid | 18:0 |
| Lignoceric acid | Tetracosanoic acid | 24:0 |
| Palmitoleic acid | *cis*-9-Hexadecenoic acid | 16:1(9) |
| Oleic acid | *cis*-9-Octadecenoic acid | 18:1(9)* |
| No name | *cis*-10-Hexadecenoic acid | 16:1(10)* |
| No name | *cis*-12-Octadecenoic acid | 18:1(12)* |
| Linoleic acid | *cis*-9,12-Octadecadienoic acid | 18:2(9,12)* |
| Linolenic acid | *cis*-9,12,15-Octadecatrienoic acid | 18:3(9,12,15) |
| Arachidonic acid | *cis*-5,8,11,14-Eicosatetraenoic acid | 20:4(5,8,11,14) |
| No name | *cis*-4,7,10,13,16,19-Docosahexaenoic acid | 22:6(4,7,10,13,16,19)† |

*Significant amounts occur as esters in precorneal tear film lipids (Nicolaides et al, 1981).

†A significant fatty acid in photoreceptor membrane phospholipids (Anderson, 1983).

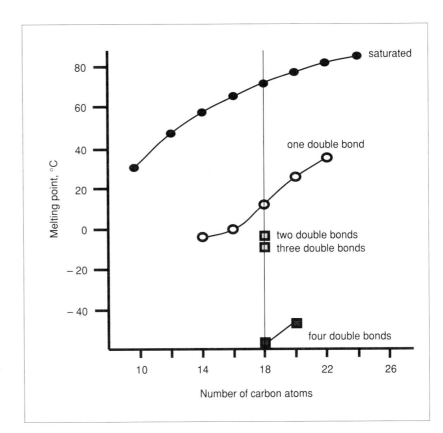

**FIGURE 4-2   The melting point of a fatty acid is an indicator of how fluid a membrane will be.**
A lower melting point is associated with greater fluidity. An increase in carbon number raises the melting point, whereas an increase in unsaturation (number of double bonds) lowers the melting point. This is most easily seen in the C-18 fatty acids designated by a vertical line.

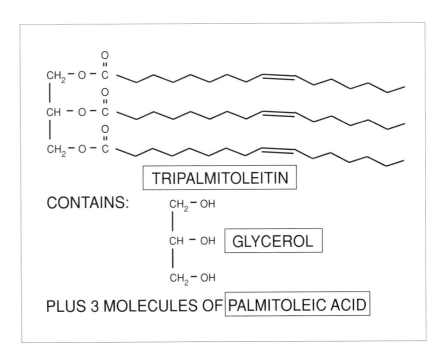

**FIGURE 4-3   Triacylglycerols are composed of glycerol and three fatty acids esterified together.**
Tripalmitoleitin is the example here. The fatty acids esterified to glycerol, however, are usually of mixed carbon numbers and saturation to maintain fluidity.

triacylglycerols but only 600 kcal in total glycogen (Stryer, 1988). The eye does not maintain any substantial reserves of lipids in the form of triacylglycerols for energy production, but does maintain a limited amount to maintain cellular membranes.

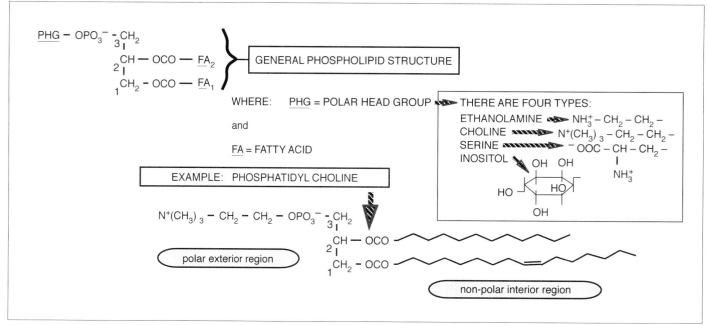

**FIGURE 4-4   The components of phospholipids.**
Phospholipids consist of glycerol, two fatty acids, and one of the four possible head groups. The fatty acids extend into the interior of a membrane, whereas the polar head group is present at the membrane-water interface.

## Phospholipids

Phospholipids are the most important lipid class for the formation and maintenance of all forms of cellular membranes. The structure of phospholipids is similar to that of triacylglycerols (see Figure 4-4 and compare with Figure 4-3). Both forms use glycerol as the "frame" on which esters are attached. In phospholipids, however, a phosphate ester is used to bond the glycerol to one of four kinds of polar groups: ethanolamine, choline (a trimethylamine), serine (the amino acid), or inositol (a polyhydroxy ring structure derived from glucose). These groups bond to C-3 of the glycerol molecule via a phosphate bridge.

Phospholipids can be made by cells in a variety of "mix-and-match" combinations. In these lipids, the fatty acid composition on C-1 and C-2 of the glycerol differs in both chain length and degree of saturation. Given the fact that the polar head groups also vary, the phospholipids are capable of existing in a great combination of both their polar and nonpolar regions. In its configuration (Figure 4-4) the charged or polar head region of the molecule protrudes into the aqueous regions (inside and outside) of a cell while the fatty acid (nonpolar) regions bury themselves in the interior of a particular membrane. Mitochondrial membranes contain another variation of phospholipid structure known as a *cardiolipin*. A cardiolipin has three glycerols esterified together on its polar region, in which the two outer glycerols are bound to four fatty acids (nonpolar region). The structure of a typical membrane with phospholipids can be seen in Figure 4-5. Note that the membrane has two lipid layers (bilayer) in which the fatty acid portions face each other (interiorly) and the polar head groups are arranged to face the aqueous portions of the inside and/or outside of a cell. The B representation in the figure was used previously in this book (see Figure 2-17).

The fatty acid composition of phospholipids in membranes is "designed" by the cell, according to its required function. For example, let us compare (Table 4-2) the fatty acid content of the phospholipid phosphatidylethanolamine in red blood cell plasma membranes with those in photoreceptor rod outer segments. The membrane of the red blood cell must be somewhat

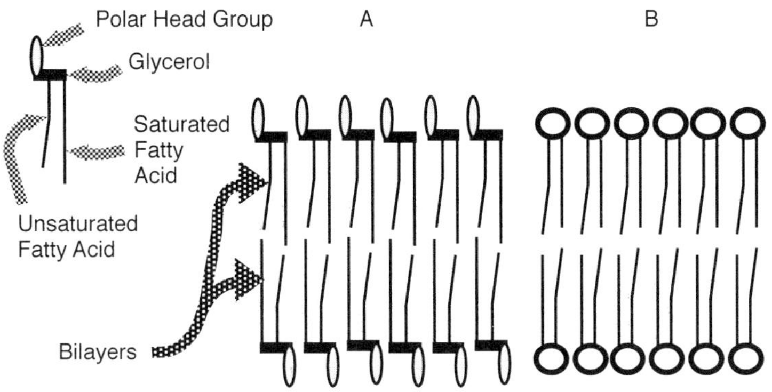

Phospholipid components (shown on the left) may be represented in a membrane as at A (above) or, more simply, as at B (above).

**FIGURE 4-5    Representations of phospholipids in a membrane.**

Scheme B is commonly used in membrane diagrams.

**TABLE 4-2    Comparative Percentage of Fatty Acids in Phosphatidylethanolamine**

| Fatty Acid | Red Blood Cell* (%) | Rod Outer Segments[†] (%) |
|---|---|---|
| 16:0 | 18 | 10 |
| 16:1 | 1 | — |
| 18:0 | 12 | 36 |
| 18:1 | 20 | 6 |
| 18:2 | 7 | — |
| 20:3 | 1 | — |
| 20:4 | 22 | 4 |
| 22:4 | 8 | — |
| 22:5 | 5 | — |
| 22:6 | 6 | 34 |
| Unknown | — | 10 |

*Red blood cell plasma membranes. Data from McGilvery and Goldstein, 1983.

[†]Rod outer segment disc membranes. Data from Anderson, 1983.

rigid to assume its biconcave disc shape. Accordingly, it tends to have more shorter-chain, unsaturated fatty acids and a smaller percentage of longer, highly unsaturated fatty acids. Rod outer segment discs, however, require a high degree of membrane fluidity to carry out the process of visual transduction, which begins with the bleaching of rhodopsin within the membrane. Therefore, the percentage of 22:6 fatty acid is almost six times greater than red blood cell plasma membranes.

## Isoprenoids

Isoprenoids are a family of lipids metabolically built up from five-carbon units each known as isoprene (Fig. 4-6, *insert*). The members include cholesterol (and its steroids), lipid-soluble vitamins such as vitamin A, coenzyme Q (discussed in Chapter 3), and other substances. Here we focus on cholesterol; later in the chapter we discuss vitamin A.

Cholesterol is a molecule composed of four fused rings, two methyl groups, a hydrocarbon branch, and a single hydroxy group. As shown it has 27 carbons (Figure 4-6). When the molecule is laid on its side, it is relatively flat, but somewhat bulky and rigid. It is a highly apolar lipid (save for the

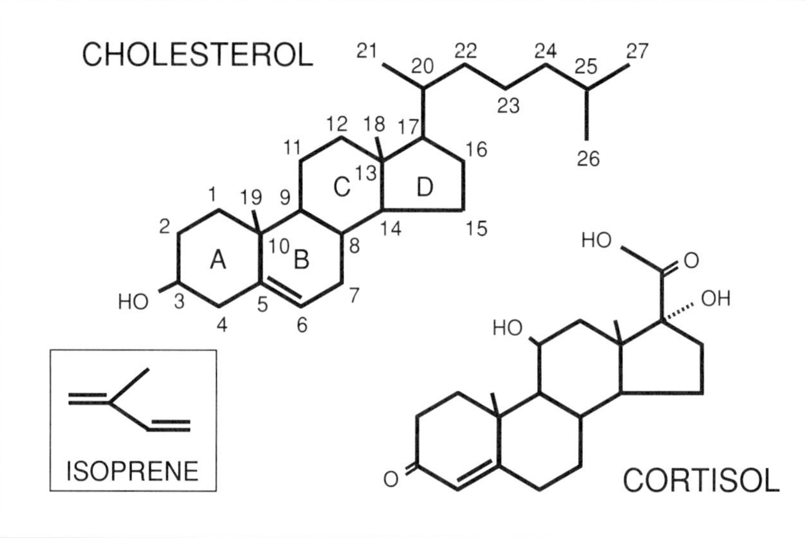

FIGURE 4-6    Two examples of isoprenoids: cholesterol and cortisol.

Cholesterol consists of 27 carbons (as numbered), of which the first 17 form four rings. Cortisol is a hormone naturally synthesized from cholesterol. Inset: an isoprene unit. It consists of five carbons with double bonds shared between four carbons. Isoprene units are building blocks of cholesterol and other isoprenoids.

single hydroxy group) and fits readily into membrane structures, where it imparts rigidity instead of fluidity to the membrane. Cholesterol is an important lipid for a variety of other reasons besides its participation in membrane rigidity. It is a source of cholesteryl esters, which are important components of the precorneal tear film. It is a synthetic precursor of a variety of steroid hormones (Chapter 6) that affect ocular function and dysfunction. Medically, there is much interest in dietary cholesterol and the deposition of cholesterol (and its esters) in blood vessels, which cause atherosclerosis and heart disease. Unfortunately, in spite of much research effort, this area remains controversial due to the complexities of cholesterol intake (diet), synthesis, transport, and metabolic relationships to the fatty acids (Mathews and van Holde, 1990).

The participation of cholesterol in membrane structures is more restricted in certain ocular membranes where fluidity is required. In fact cholesterol makes up only 10% of the lipids of rod outer segment membranes of retinal photoreceptors (Anderson, 1983).

The detection of cholesterol in tissues has also been used to determine disease origin. For example, a disease known as chalazion, which is a granulomatous inflammation of the eyelid margin, was formerly associated with meibomian gland lipids. However, the lipids determined in chalazia are rich in cholesterol (a membrane lipid) rather than cholesteryl esters (meibomian gland lipids) (Nicolaides et al., 1988). Accordingly, it was concluded that the meibomian gland does not cause the disease, since the source of this lipid is actually the membranes of the neutrophils, lymphocytes, and other white blood cells that bring about the inflammation.

### Esters

Esters are a general class of lipids, but also are the name of the bonds formed between a carboxylic acid (which is what a fatty acid is) and either an alcohol (derived from a fatty acid) or a hydroxy group attached to a ring compound (both aromatic and nonaromatic types) that occur in this class. Examples of lipid esters have already been seen with bonds formed between glycerol and fatty acids in the formation of triacylglycerols (see Figure 4-3) and phospholipids (see Figure 4-4). In addition, the hydroxy group of cholesterol forms cholesteryl esters with fatty acids (Figure 4-7). The

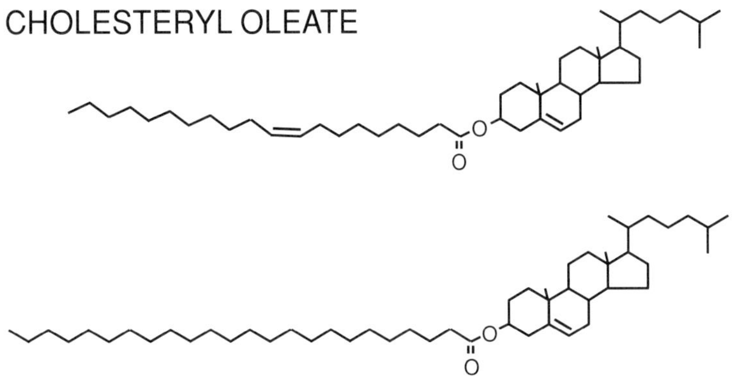

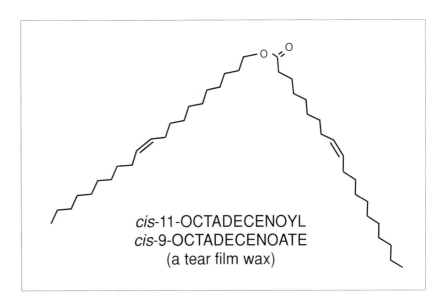

**FIGURE 4-7** Two cholesteryl esters formed from cholesterol and a fatty acid. Cholesteryl pentacosate is a tear film lipid.

second example in the figure contains an odd-numbered fatty acid peculiar to precorneal tear film cholesteryl esters. A third type of lipid ester is represented by waxes, esters of long-chain (14 to 36-carbon) fatty acids and long-chain (16 to 20-carbon) alcohols derived from fatty acids. Waxes are usually solid at room temperature and occur, in nature, as the shiny covering of plant leaves, the substance known as beeswax, and the oily substances that cover skin, hair, wool, and animal fur. In the eye, waxes are a major component of the lipid layer of the precorneal tear film (Figure 4-8).

## Eicosanoids

Eicosanoids are cyclic lipids derived from eicosanoic (20-carbon) acids such as arachidonic acid. They include prostaglandins, thromboxanes, and leukotrienes. An example may be found in Figure 4-9. The eicosanoids are short-acting local hormones, considered in Chapter 6.

## Glycolipids

Glycolipids (Figure 4-9) are important membrane components found in nervous, ocular, and other tissues. Glycolipids, as their name implies, are

**FIGURE 4-8** Another tear film lipid, a wax. It is made up of a fatty acid and a fatty acid alcohol. The first substance (*cis*-11-octadecenoyl) is the alcohol.

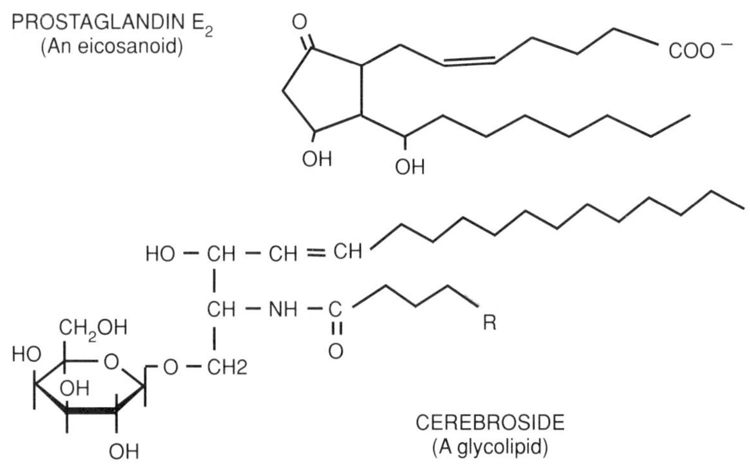

FIGURE 4-9  An example of an eicosanoid (prostaglandin E₂) and a glycolipid (cerebroside).

lipids that contain carbohydrates such as galactose, $N$-acetylgalactose, and a derivative known as $N$-acetylneuraminic acid (sialic acid, Figure 4-10). The basic structure that hinges glycolipids together is not glycerol but a long-chain amino alcohol known as *sphingosine* (Figure 4-11). It resembles glycerol, but has a single fatty acid derivative permanently attached to it as well as an amino group. When a second fatty acid is bound to sphingosine the compound is known as a *ceramide*. When phosphocholine is esterified to the ceramide, the compound becomes *sphingomyelin* (Figure 4-12). If the phosphocholine is replaced by one or more carbohydrates, the compound becomes a *glycolipid* (or more precisely, a *glycosphingolipid*) such as the cerebroside and the ganglioside in Figures 4-12, 4-13.

The particular ganglioside shown in Figure 4-13 is known as $G_{M2}$ or Tay-Sachs ganglioside. It is, however, actually a partially degraded ganglioside that accumulates in neural, ocular, and other tissues in the course of Tay-Sachs disease. The disease occurs as a result of a deficiency of the enzyme hexosaminidase A, which normally catalyzes the turnover (breakdown) of old $G_{M2}$ molecules while new molecules are synthesized. As a result of the accumulation of $G_{M2}$ in the retina, the ganglion cells degenerate, producing

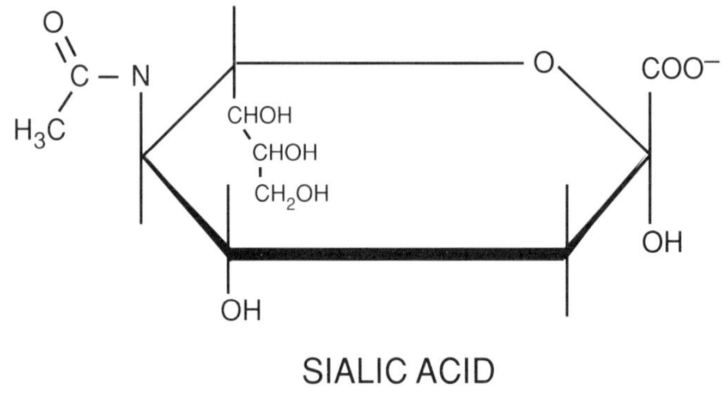

FIGURE 4-10  Sialic acid or *N*-acetylneuraminic acid.
This is a complex, modified carbohydrate found on glycolipids and glycoproteins. One role of sialic acid is to prevent the oligosaccharide chain from binding to surface receptors of other cells.

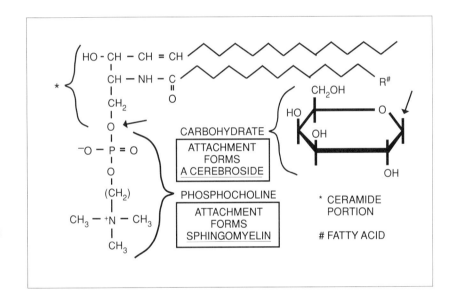

SPHINGOSINE
(The glycolipid "hinge" molecule)

**IGURE 4-11** The sphingosine molecule.
phingosine is used in place of glycerol to form glycolipids
nd sphingomyelin. This molecule has a long chain
ydrocarbon (derived from a fatty acid) and an amino
roup in place of one hydroxy group.

**IGURE 4-12 A combined example of a cerebroside (a
glycolipid having one carbohydrate) and
phingomyelin.**
The arrows show the point of binding between the
galactose and the ceremide moieties.

a characteristic cherry-red spot in the macular region (Libert and Kenyon, 1986). Unfortunately this condition results in blindness at a very early age. It is also accompanied by arrested motor and mental development. Patients usually die between 3 to 6 years of age (Brady, 1982). Tay-Sachs disease is one of a number of metabolic storage diseases that involve an enzyme defect (or deficiency) in the catabolism of GAGs or glycolipids. An example was given in Chapter 3. These diseases generally affect either the cornea (producing cloudiness) or the retina (producing degenerative blindness). Each disease is inherited, but, fortunately, they are comparatively rare (Grayson, 1979).

## Cell Membranes

Cellular membranes are such important functional barriers that some additional comments are necessary. Membranes must ultimately be considered as walls built up of lipids, carbohydrates, and proteins. Up to now consideration has been fixed on the lipid components, since they are the major

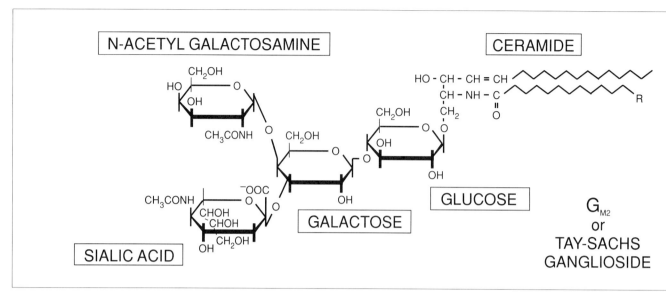

**FIGURE 4-13   The Tay-Sachs ganglioside.**
This is a partially degraded ganglioside. The complete, in situ, ganglioside, known as $G_{M1}$, has a galactose attached to N-acetylgalactosamine, which is detached by β-galactosidase in neural and ocular cell lysosomes. In Tay-Sachs disease, the N-acetylgalactosamine (which would normally be hydrolyzed next) is not removed, due to a deficiency of the enzyme hexosaminidase.

components. The carbohydrate components, as with the gangliosides just considered, have functions that are directed predominantly toward the exterior side of cells. These roles include the anchoring and orientation of plasma membrane proteins, cell recognition (e.g., immunological identification: friend or foe), cell-cell identification and interaction, as well as interaction with noncellular matrices such as collagenous basement membranes. Cells are, in fact, often surrounded by dense carbohydrate branches that are anchored in the membranes. These branches form the outer coat, or *glycocalyx*, of cells. Some carbohydrates are directed toward the interior of membrane compartments. In the eye, an example of such an internally directed glycoprotein-containing membrane is in photoreceptor outer segment discs (see Figure 1-16). There the oligosaccharides attached to rhodopsin are located on the intradiscal side of the membrane.

The protein components of membranes fall into two categories: intrinsic or integral (located within the bilipid layer), and extrinsic or peripheral (located on or attached to one hydrophilic surface of the membrane). *Intrinsic membrane proteins* tend to have operational roles: transport (e.g., of glucose), reception (e.g., of insulin), transduction (e.g., of light), and attachment (e.g., to basement membranes). *Peripheral proteins* usually have more passive roles: structural (e.g., cytoskeleton maintenance), anchoring (e.g., for glycocalyx components), and cell local movement (e.g., myosin and actin components). The transport of substances across cell boundaries may or may not include transport proteins.

Three general types of transport are recognized: simple diffusion, passive transport, and active transport. In simple diffusion, very small molecules such as water and hydrophobic gases readily cross membranes (going from an area of higher concentration to one of lower concentration). In passive or facilitated transport, a protein acts as a gate or channel to assist a substance (such as $Na^+$ or $K^+$) in crossing the membrane (again, going from an area of higher concentration to one of lower concentration). In active transport, a protein enzyme moves a substance (such as glucose) from an area of *lower to higher* concentration. Any form of protein-assisted transport is rate limited (only so many molecules can be transported at a maximal rate). As with enzyme kinetics, such transport is subject to competition or inhibition.

Our current knowledge of membrane structure and function is based on the hypothesis of Singer and Nicholson (1972). A composite illustration of all the kinds of components of a cell membrane is shown in Figure 4-14, and there are many other examples throughout this book. Finally, it is important to understand that lipid variations are introduced by cells into their membrane components. This is done to obtain optimal usage of the membrane for the well-being of the cell. For example, the bilipid layers of membranes are asymmetric. This means that the phospholipid composition varies on each side of the membrane. In red blood cells approximately 75% of the phosphatidylcholine is located on the exterior bilipid layer, whereas 80% of the phosphatidylethanolamine is on the interior layer (Houslay and Stanley, 1982). It is generally true that choline-containing phospholipids predominate on the outer bilipid layer, along with cholesterol. This asymmetry helps the membrane assume a certain amount of curvature. The total lipid, protein, and carbohydrate composition of membranes also varies with membrane type (Table 4-3).

## Precorneal Tear Film Lipids

When tears are spread across the cornea after eyelid blinking, the thinned-out liquid that results is called the *precorneal tear film*. The layer consists of three parts. The most anterior or superficial lipid layer is 0.1 μm thick. This covers a 7-μm aqueous layer, which in turn covers a 0.002 to 0.005-μm mucus layer. The latter is properly described as a protein coating on top of the epithelial cells. The aqueous layer contains a variety of dissolved salts and proteins. The lipid layer consists predominately of a large variety of waxes and cholesteryl esters whose general structural characteristics were mentioned previously. Tears (and the tear film) represent a protective coating for the outer surface of the eye. The tears wash away debris from the corneal surface and, therefore, act as a perfusion fluid. The tear film is an optically uniform surface and contains lysozyme (Chapter 2) and other proteins that possess antibacterial functions (Milder, 1987). The lipid layer of the film serves the basic function of stabilizing the period of time in which the film remains intact (15 to 40 seconds) before it ruptures and stimulates the next blink (Davson, 1990).

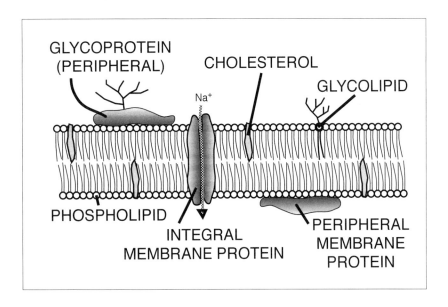

**FIGURE 4-14** The common lipid, protein, and carbohydrate components of cell plasma membranes. Note that the carbohydrate components are always bound to either a lipid or a protein.

**TABLE 4-3  Percentage Composition (by Weight) of Membrane Components**

| Membrane Source | Lipid | Protein | Carbohydra |
|---|---|---|---|
| Red blood cell | 43 | 49 | 8 |
| Myelin sheath | 79 | 18 | 3 |
| Mitochondrion (outer membrane) | 47 | 51 | 2 |
| Mitochondrion (inner membrane) | 23 | 76 | 1 |
| Bovine retinal rods | 47 | 49 | 4 |

(Adapted from Guidotti G. Membrane proteins. *Ann Rev Biochem* 1972;41:732.

**TABLE 4-4  Composition of Human Meibomian Gland Lipids**

| Lipid Component | Composition (% |
|---|---|
| Cholesteryl esters | 29.5 |
| Wax esters | 35 |
| Triacylglycerols | 4 |
| Cholesterol | 1.8 |
| Fatty acids | 2.2 |
| Unidentified* | 27.5 |

*These unidentified components can be further subdivided on the basis of their polar/nonpo
lar properties. Some have been recently identified (see text).

(Nicolaides N. In Holly FJ (ed). *The Precorneal Tear Film in Health, Disease, and Contact Lens Wea*
Lubbock, TX: Dry Eye Institute, 1986;573.)

**TABLE 4-5  Fatty Acids in the Precorneal Tear Film**

| Fatty Acid Characteristic | Numbe |
|---|---|
| Carbon length (all types) | 14–36 C |
| Number of double bonds | 0–3 |
| Hydroxy straight chain length | 29–36 C |
| Hydroxy branched chain (number of carbons) | 29–34 C |

*Includes odd numbered lengths which are comparatively rare in animal tissues.

†Values given for cattle. Human values are similar.

(Nicolaides N. Recent findings on the chemical composition of the lipids of steer and huma
meibomian glands. *In* Holly FJ (ed). *The Precorneal Tear Film in Health, Disease, and Contact Len*
*Wear.* Lubbock, TX: Dry Eye Institute, 1986;570–596.)

The composition of lipids in the tears is complex. A large variety of fatty
acids, their alcohol derivatives, and cholesterol make up the waxes and
cholesteryl esters found there. Other lipid classes are also present (Nico
laides 1986) (Table 4-4). Slightly more than 25% of the lipid types have no
been completely characterized. They include 8.4% double esters or diester
(Figure 4-15) in which hydroxy fatty acids are esterified to two other fatty
acids or an alcohol or a cholesterol molecule. Four percent of the lipid
represent uncombined, precursor fatty acids and cholesterol molecules
The varieties of fatty acids are listed in Table 4-5. Nicolaides (1986) ha
estimated that, with some 69 different fatty acids, 40 fatty acid alcohols, and
11 hydroxy fatty acids in meibomian gland secretions, about 30,000 este
species are possible. The cooperative physicochemical properties of these
esters render lipids capable of (1) flowing from their ducts to the eyelic
edges, (2) forming a film over the aqueous layer and maintaining contac

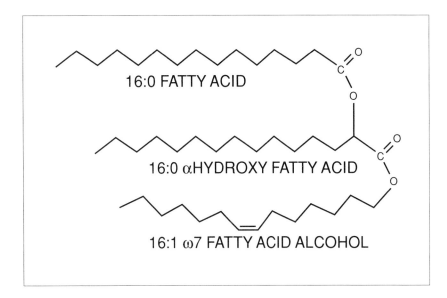

**FIGURE 4-15   A diester component of the lipid layer of the precorneal tear film.**
Here the diester is composed of a fatty acid, a hydroxy fatty acid, and a long-chain alcohol (fatty acid alcohol).

with it, (3) adhering to the eyelid skin and acting as a barrier to the aqueous layer, and (4) forming a watertight seal when the lids are closed.

Pathological conditions can alter this exquisite ester mixture and bring about tear film abnormalities. In meibomian gland dysfunction, for example, excessive production of keratin occurs in the ductal epithelium. Keratin is a protein characteristic of skin and hard coverings such as animal horns. Nicolaides et al. (1989) have suggested that this process alters the composition of tear film lipids to include the lipid composition of the keratinized epithelial cells, composed of decreased steryl esters, increased cholesterol, and increased ceramides. A further complication of this process is that the epithelial cells detach from the gland and block the flow of lipids to the tear film. This alone causes more rapid breakup of the tear film. Still another alteration that may accompany these events is bacterial infection in the area of the blocked lipids. McCulley and Dougherty (1986) have shown that *Staphylococcus aureus* and other bacteria produce a cholesteryl esterase and a fatty wax esterase that are capable of hydrolyzing the meibomian lipids.

## Lipids of the Retina

In the retina, photoreceptors, together with other neural cells, operate the complete transduction mechanism for converting light energy into electrical signaling and sending the signals to the brain. The phospholipid-fatty acid composition of the retinal membrane lipids is shown in Table 4-6. Compare the phosphatidylethanolamine fatty acid composition in Table 4-6 with that for photoreceptors in Table 4-2. The compositions, taken from two independent investigations, are virtually the same, showing that the percentages of fatty acids in both retina and photoreceptor membranes are similar. That is, they have a high concentration of 22:6. It is also worth pointing out that the percentages of phospholipids resemble those of nervous tissue (Broekhuyse and Daemen, 1977). However, the phospholipids in photoreceptors have less sphingomyelin and phosphatidylinositol.

The lipid content of rod and cone outer segments is quite high because of the presence of the discs. These discs are separated by a distance of only

**TABLE 4-6   Phospholipid and Fatty Acid Composition of Mammalian Retina**

| *Phospholipid Composition* * (%) | | *Fatty Acid Composition* * (%) | | | | |
|---|---|---|---|---|---|---|
| *Type* | *%* | *16:0* | *18:0* | *18:1* | *20:4* | *22:6* |
| Phosphatidylcholine | 41 | 41 | 18 | 18 | 5 | 11 |
| Phosphatidylethanolamine | 34 | 10 | 32 | 8 | 8 | 29 |
| Phosphatidylserine | 10 | 6 | 34 | 15 | 3 | 24 |
| Phosphatidylinositol | 6 | 7 | 36 | 7 | 42 | 3 |
| Sphingomyelin | 4 | 25 | 42 | 11 | <1 | <1 |

*Since some types are not presented percentages do not total 100%.

(Broekhuyse RM, and Daemen FJM. The eye. In Snyder F (ed). *Lipid Metabolism in Mammals*. New York: Plenum Press, 1977; 161.

300 Å. The lipid composition is 15% of the wet weight of a rod outer segment. By comparison, the lipid content of most cells is only about 1%. The high concentration of docosahexaenoic acid (22:6) in photoreceptors, mentioned under fatty acids correlates with the low viscosity of photoreceptor membrane discs. That is, the high fluidity of the discs contributes to the important rotational and lateral movements of rhodopsin. Moreover, there seems to be a preservation mechanism for this fatty acid, since the reduction of essential fatty acids in the diets of laboratory animals has no effect on reducing the amount of 22:6 in their retinas. Essential fatty acids are precursors of 22:6. Polyunsaturated fatty acids such as 22:6 are vulnerable to destruction by oxidative processes in the retina (Broekhuyse and Daemen 1977); however, Anderson (1983) has suggested that there are sufficient concentrations of vitamin E there to prevent such destruction. Vitamin E or α-tocopherol (Figure 4-16) acts by absorbing free radicals (unpaired electrons) that are found in active forms of oxygen and hydroxide radicals. If vitamin E were not present, such free radicals would attack the double bonds of membrane fatty acids (such as 22:6) and break them up into fragmentary aldehydes (Mayes, 1985).

## Vitamin A

In Chapter 1, we discussed the linkage of 11-*cis* vitamin A aldehyde, or retinal, to opsin to form rhodopsin. Vitamin A is a hydrophobic vitamin that belongs to the isoprenoid class of lipids. It is also called a fat-soluble vitamin. The dietary sources of vitamin A are β-carotene (Figure 4-17) and retinyl

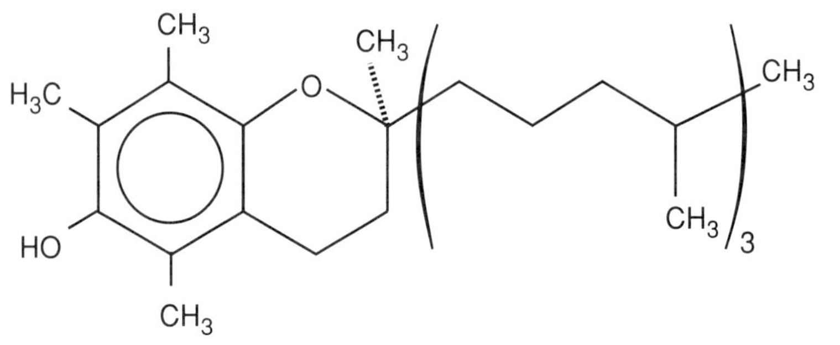

**FIGURE 4-16   Vitamin E (α-tocopherol).**
An isoprenoid lipid with vitamin properties, it is also an antioxidant. It acts by absorbing highly reactive, unpaired electrons into the resonance system of the left-hand ring.

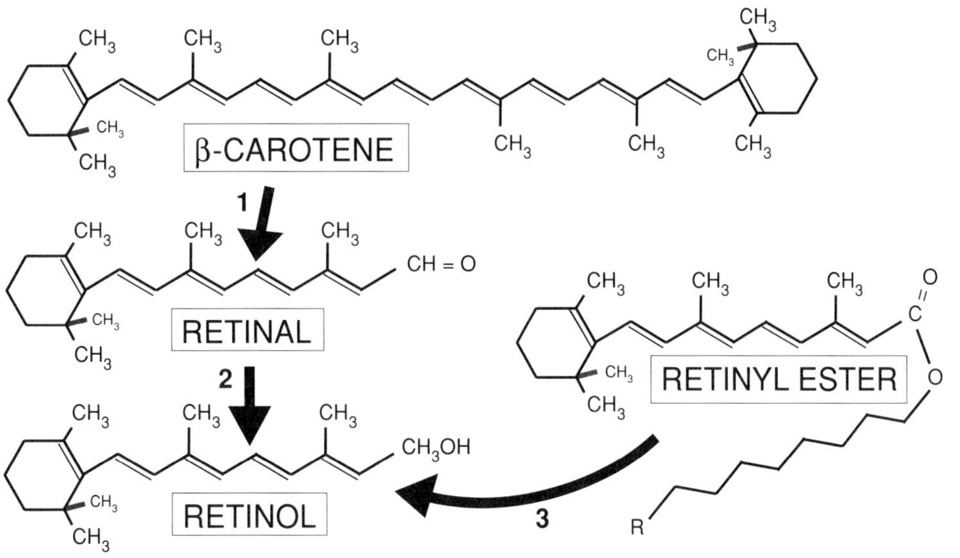

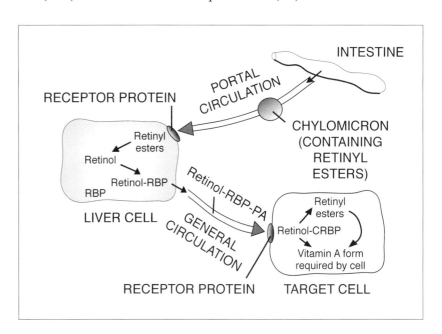

β-CAROTENE

RETINAL

RETINYL ESTER

RETINOL

**FIGURE 4-17  Dietary forms of vitamin A are β-carotene (actually a precursor of vitamin A) and retinyl ester.**
In the intestines, β-carotene is broken into two retinal molecules by β-carotene dioxygenase (reaction 1) with the aid of molecular oxygen and bile salts (cholesterol derivatives). The retinal is reduced to retinol with retinol reductase (reaction 2) using NADPH as a coenzyme. Retinyl ester is hydrolyzed to retinol with an esterase (reaction 3). The retinol is absorbed into the intestinal cells and, incredibly, reesterified again with long-chain saturated fatty acids for incorporation into chylomicra.

esters. The former occurs in yellow vegetables such as carrots and sweet potatoes whereas the latter comes from animal sources (Lehninger, 1982). In the gut both sources are enzymatically converted, predominately to retinol or vitamin A alcohol (Figure 4-18). Some retinoic acid is also formed. The retinol becomes reesterified and is incorporated into chylomicra for transport to the liver. Chylomicra are lipid spheres in which the more hydrophobic lipids are incorporated interiorly and the more hydrophilic lipids coat the surface of the sphere, where they are complexed with proteins. Chylomicra are transport complexes that are compatible with the aqueous environment of the bloodstream. Vitamin A transport is principally to the liver, where reesterification and storage occur.

When needed, mobilization of vitamin A, largely in the form of retinol, takes place after binding the vitamin to two proteins: retinol-binding protein (RBP) inside the cell and then prealbumin (PA) in the bloodstream. In

**FIGURE 4-18  The processing and transport of vitamin A to its target cells.**
Key: RBP, retinol-binding protein; PA, prealbumin; CRBP, cellular retinol-binding protein. CRBP is used to bind retinol only inside cells.

this complex form retinol is transported through the bloodstream to it target cells such as the pigmented epithelial cells of the retina and the corneal epithelial cells. Upon reaching its target cell, retinol is released an transported via a receptor protein (Chader, 1982) into the cell cytoplasm There, as in the liver, it may be stored as an ester after binding to a cellula retinol binding protein (CRBP) or converted to a useful form for the ce These actions, to this point, are shown in Figure 4-18.

It should be apparent by now that there are several chemical forms c vitamin A. These are summarized (Table 4-7). These forms have many role besides support of visual transduction. Retinol functions as a hormone, i addition to being a transport form, in order to control protein synthesis. W take this up again in Chapter 6. Retinoic acid is involved in both the forma tion of glycoproteins and the maturation of epithelial cells, including thos in the corneal epithelium. Retinal, as the 11-*cis* form, binds to opsin to forr rhodopsin, as discussed in Chapter 1. Figure 4-19 shows the sequence c events between the pigment epithelial cells and the photoreceptors tha leads to the formation of 11-*cis* retinal.

Most of the scientific knowledge of the functions of vitamin A has bee gained from observing what happens to ocular and nonocular tissues as result of vitamin A deficiency. An early effect is the loss of night visio (nyctalopia). This is followed by hardening of the corneal conjunctiva wit the loss of conjunctival secretions (xerophthalmia or dry eye), and eventu ally keratomalacia (degeneration of the cornea) may develop. The latte condition may ultimately result in corneal perforation. Although rare in th United States, homeless people, the elderly and others on a poor diet ma develop some of these symptoms over time. Vitamin A–related ocular symp toms are common in nations with poor vitamin A diets. Nonocular symptom generally include adverse effects in any tissues covered by epithelial cel and inhibition of bone elongation. Children are, therefore, particularl subject to growth retardation from vitamin A deficiency.

Vitamin A, unfortunately, also has adverse effects when taken exces sively. The normal FDA daily recommended intake is given in Table 4-8 Americans have become so vitamin conscious that they sometimes tend t exceed the recommended amounts, figuring that more is better; howeve Hathcock et al. (1990) have shown that when the daily intake of this vitami exceeds 10,000 IU, adverse symptoms begin to appear: abdominal pair

**TABLE 4-7   Chemical Forms of Vitamin A and Their Roles**

| Name | Form | Role(s) |
|---|---|---|
| Retinyl ester | Vitamin—$CH_2$—O—$\overset{\overset{O}{\|\|}}{C}$—fatty acid | Storage |
| Retinol | Vitamin—$CH_2$—OH | Transport, hormonal |
| Retinal | Vitamin—CH=O[†] | Visual transduction |
| Retinoic acid | Vitamin—C—OH ($\overset{\|\|}{O}$) | Synthesis[‡] |

*Acts at the cell nucleus to influence gene expression.

[†]Exists as the 11-*cis* form (see Figure 1-17). All other forms are the all-*trans* isomers.

[‡]Acts as an agent in the synthesis of glycoproteins and in the differentiation of all types c epithelial cells.

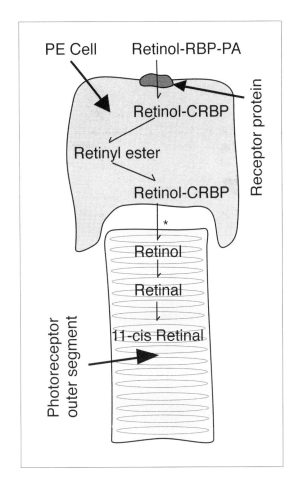

**FIGURE 4-19** The processing and transport of vitamin A at pigment epithelial (PE) cells and photoreceptor outer segments.

At PE cells retinol may be stored as an ester or transported to the outer segment. The transport between PE cell and photoreceptor outer segment of retinol (*) seems to make use of another binding protein, an interstitial retinol binding protein (IRBP), as described by Hollyfield et al (1985). In the outer segment, retinol is converted to retinal (still in the all-*trans* form) and then to 11-*cis* retinal. Whether or not enzyme-catalyzed reactions are involved does not seem to have been resolved (Shichi, 1983).

**TABLE 4-8   U.S. Food and Drug Administration Recommended Daily Allowance (RDA) of Vitamin A**

| Group | RDA (IU)* |
|---|---|
| Infants ($\leq$ 12 mo) | 1500 |
| Children ($<$ 4 y) | 2500 |
| Childen ($>$ 4 y) to Adults | 5000 |
| Lactating or pregnant women | 8000 |

*IU = international units. 1 IU = 0.3 $\mu$g retinol. For an adult this is equal to 1.5 mg retinol.

blurred vision, drowsiness, headache, irritability, nausea, and vomiting. Two biochemical aspects of excessive vitamin A intake are increased gluconeogenesis and protein turnover. Other than blurred vision, however, excessive vitamin A intake does not seem to have any other ocular effects.

## Summary

Although predominately hydrophobic, lipids have hydrophilic regions that allow them to interact with aqueous media. This amphipathic characteristic of lipids is ideal for their important role in defining cell boundaries as membranes. Lipids also function as hormones, sources of energy, and as an important part of visual transduction. There are seven major lipid classe[ fatty acids, triacylglycerols, phospholipids, isoprenoids, esters, eicosanoid and glycolipids. The lipids that make up cell membranes vary in compos tion to suit the requirements of particular cells. In photoreceptor discs, fc example, a high percentage of docosahexaenoic acid (22:6) is used to mair tain maximal fluidity of the membrane. The precorneal tear film lipids cor sist largely of waxes and cholesteryl esters. This unique and comple mixture ensures optimal spreading and stability of the tear film. Vitami A is important for ocular function in two ways. First, it combines wit opsin, forming rhodopsin, in the form of 11-*cis* retinal. This holoprotei reacts with light to initiate visual transduction. Second, it maintains th proper development of corneal epithelial and conjunctival tissues. A lack c vitamin A in the diet can lead to night blindness and keratinization of th cornea.

## References

Anderson RE. Chemistry of photoreceptor outer segments. *In* Anderson R (ed). *Biochemistry of the Eye.* San Francisco: American Academy of Ophthal mology, 1983;166–167.

Brady RO. Sphingolipidoses and other lipid metabolic disorders. *In* Siege GJ, Albers RW, Agranoff BW, and Katzman R (eds). *Basic Neurochemistr*y 3rd ed. Boston: Little, Brown, 1982;622.

Broekhuyse RM, and Daemen FJM. The eye. *In* Synder F (ed). *Lipid Metab olism in Mammals.* New York: Plenum Press, 1977;161.

Chader GJ. Retinoids in ocular tissues: Binding proteins, transport, an mechanism of action. *In* McDevitt DS (ed). *Cell Biology of the Eye.* Nev York: Academic Press, 1982;377–433.

Davson H. *Physiology of the Eye,* 5th ed. New York: Pergamon Press, 199C 792–794.

Grayson M. *Diseases of the Cornea.* St. Louis; CV Mosby, 1979;396–415.

Hathcock JN, Hattan DG, Jenkins MY, McDonald JT, Sundaresan PR, an Wilkening VL. Evaluation of vitamin A toxicity. *Am J Clin Nut* 1990;52:183–202.

Hollyfield, JG, Fliesler SJ, Rayborn ME, Fong S-L, Landers RA, and Bridge CD. Synthesis and secretion of interstitial retinol binding protein by th human retina. *Invest Ophthalmol Vis Sci* 1985;26:58–67.

Houslay MD, and Stanley KK. *Dynamics of Biological Membranes.* New York John Wiley and Sons, 1982;179.

Lehninger AL. *Principles of Biochemistry.* New York: Worth, 1982; 774.

Libert J, and Kenyon KR. Ocular ultrastructure in inborn lysosomal storag diseases. *In* Reine WA (ed). *Goldberg's Genetic and Metabolic Eye Diseas* Boston: Little, Brown & Co., 1986;111–138.

Mathews CK, and van Holde KE. *Biochemistry.* Redwood City, CA: Ben jamin/Cummings, 1990;621–631.

Mayes PA. Lipids. *In* Martin DW, Mayes OA, Rodwell VW, and Granne DK. *Harper's Review of Biochemistry,* 20th ed. Los Altos, CA: Lange Medical 1985;204-205.

McCulley JP, and Dougherty JM. Meibomian lipids in chronic blepharitis. *In* Holly FJ (ed). *The Precorneal Tear Film in Health, Disease, and Contact Lens Wear.* Lubbock, TX: Dry Eye Institute, 1986;626–631.

McGilvery RW, and Goldstein GW. *Biochemistry: A Functional Approach,* 3rd ed. Philadelphia: WB Saunders, 1983;218.

Milder B. The lacrimal apparatus. *In* Moses RE and Hart WM (eds). *Adler's Physiology of the Eye.* St. Louis: CV Mosby, 1987;15–21.

Nicolaides N. Recent findings on the chemical composition of the lipids of steer and human meibomian glands. *In* Holly FJ (ed). *The Precorneal Tear Film in Health, Disease, and Contact Lens Wear.* Lubbock, TX: Dry Eye Institute, 1986;570–596.

Nicolaides N, Flores A, Santos EC, Robin JB, and Smith RE. The lipids of chalazia. *Invest Ophthalmol Vis Sci* 1988;29:482–486.

Nicolaides N, Kaitaranta JK, Rawdah TN, Macy JI, Boswell FM, and Smith RE. Meibomian gland studies. Comparison of steer and human lipids. *Invest Opthalmol Vis Science* 1981;20:522–536.

Nicolaides N, Santose EC, Smith RE, and Jester JV. Meibomian gland dysfunction. III: Meibomian gland lipids. *Invest Ophthalmol Vis Sci* 1989;30:946–951.

Shichi H. *Biochemistry of Vision.* New York: Academic Press, 1983;122–142.

Singer SJ, and Nicolson GL. The fluid mosaic model of the structure of cell membranes. *Science* 1972;175:720–731.

Skelton WP, and Skelton NK. Deficiency of vitamins A, B and C. *Postgrad Med* 1990;87(4):273–310.

Stryer L. *Biochemistry.* New York: WH Freeman, 1988;471.

———. National Research Council. Recommended Dietary Allowances, 9th ed. Washington, DC: Food and Nutrition Board, National Academy of Sciences, 1980.

# Chapter 5

# Nucleic Acids

Molecular biology, or nucleic acid biochemistry, is one of the most rapidly growing areas of biological research, due to both the importance of the roles of nucleic acids and the technological developments of this area. Both multicellular and unicellular organisms rely on the operations of nucleic acids to determine growth, division, function, development, and hereditary characteristics. In addition, the control and reactivity of nucleic acids are central to bacterial and viral infections, as is the uncontrolled cellular division that we know by the general term: cancer. There are also many metabolic diseases that can be traced to enzyme defects caused by some hereditary problem. Nucleic acids have two principal biochemical functions: to maintain the code for the amino acid sequence of thousands of cellular proteins and to synthesize those proteins. The functions of nucleic acids in the eye have only recently come under scrutiny, but already some rather interesting information has been obtained.

## Review of Nucleic Acid Biochemistry

### Deoxyribonucleic Acid

Two forms of nucleic acids are found in nature: deoxyribonucleic acid (DNA) and ribonucleic acid (RNA). DNA is the nucleic acid form that preserves the code for making all the proteins needed by a cell. RNA translates that code into specific proteins. DNA and RNA have certain chemical attributes in common. They are polymers of nitrogen-containing bases (adenine, guanine, cytosine, and thymine [or, in RNA, uracil]) that are joined together by sugar phosphates (Figure 5-1).

When the pentoses deoxyribose (DNA) and ribose (in RNA) are each joined to a base, the compound is known as a *nucleoside*, and the bases are adenosine, guanosine, cytidine, and thymidine(or, in RNA, uridine) respectively. The prefix *deoxy* is used if the sugar is a deoxypentose. In this case, the 2' hydroxy group is replaced by hydrogen. When a phosphopentose, such as deoxyribose phosphate, is joined to a base, the compound is known as a *nucleotide*, and the bases, as just given, add the word phosphate to their name: e.g., deoxyadenosine 5'-triphosphate, adenosine 5'-triphosphate (ATP), guanosine 3',5'-monophosphate (also known as cyclic GMP, see Chapter 6), and deoxycytidine 5'-monophosphate (Figure 5-2). Only the first example would be incorporated into a molecule of DNA. The second example may act either as a source of cellular energy (see Chapter 3) or be incorporated into a molecule of RNA. Cyclic GMP, the third example, acts as an intracellular hormone and deoxycytidine 5'-monophosphate, the fourth example, is a breakdown product of DNA.

The 2'-deoxynucleotides of the four bases (see Figure 5-1) are the only nucleotides incorporated into DNA. In order to be incorporated they must first exist in the triphosphate form. They become bound to DNA by the catalytic activity of a polymerase enzyme. In the process, a diphosphate group is *removed* from the deoxynucleotide triphosphate. Synthesis proceeds with the addition of the 5' phosphate end of the added nucleotide to the 3' end of the growing chain (Figure 5-3).

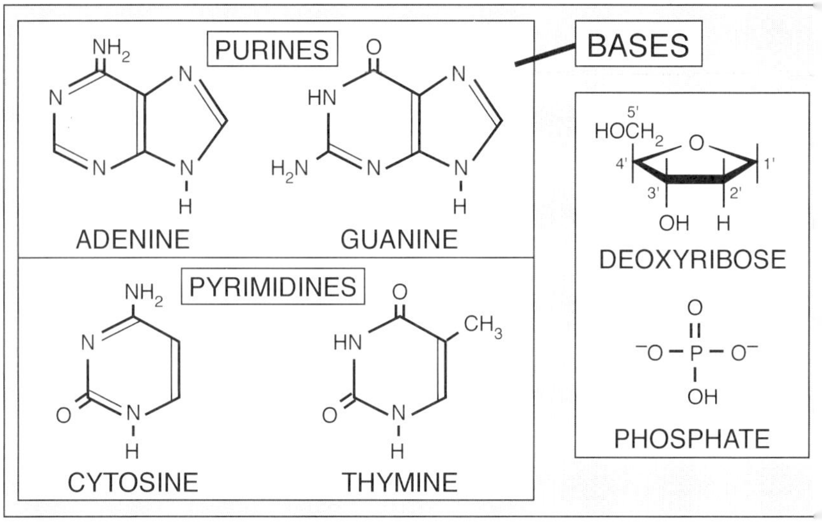

**FIGURE 5-1   The chemical components of nucleic acids.**
The bases (heterocyclic rings containing nitrogen) consist of two purines and two pyrimidines. In RNA, thymine is replaced by uracil and deoxyribose by ribose (see Figure 5-10).

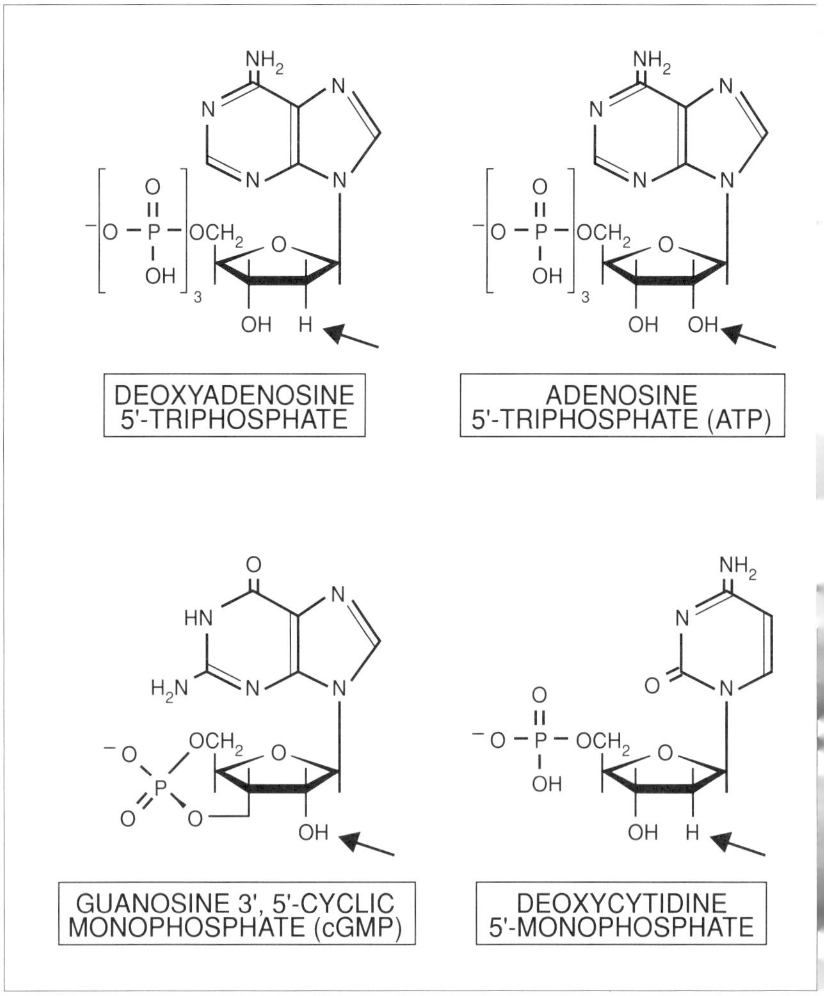

**FIGURE 5-2   Four examples of nucleotides.**
The two triphosphates at the top are precursors for incorporation into DNA (*left*) and RNA (*right*). The bottom example (*left*) is not incorporated into nucleic acids but serves as an internal hormone (see Chapter 6). The bottom example (*right*) is a breakdown product of DNA. The arrows indicate whether each example is hydroxylated or not in the 2' position of the pentose.

Several features of the DNA chain (Figure 5-3) should be noted. The DNA, once made, is double-stranded in *eukaryotes* (cells that have a nucleus). The bases are held together by hydrogen bonds: two bonds between adenine (A) and thymine (T), and three between guanine (G) and cytosine

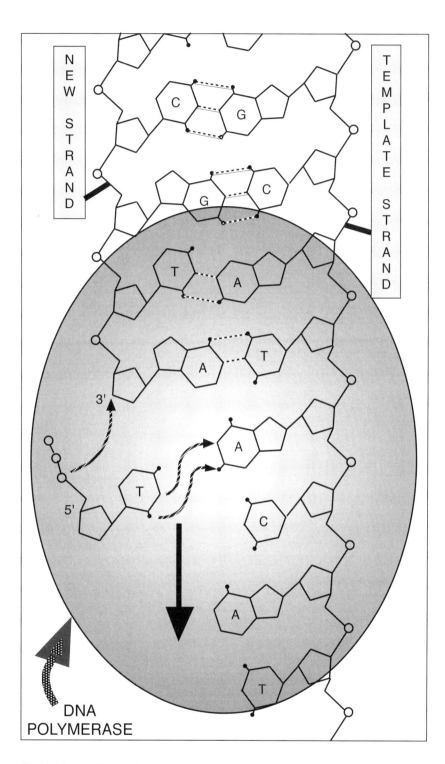

**FIGURE 5-3   DNA replication by DNA-directed DNA polymerase.**

The enzyme forms 5′→3′ bonds with each incorporated base. Hydrogen bonds (A—T), (G—C) form spontaneously after 5′→3′ bonding where the black and white lines are shown. Each triphosphate nucleotide loses a diphosphate group in the catalytic process. The base to be added is determined by the complementary, opposite base on the template strand.

(C). The bases themselves are relatively hydrophobic, whereas the deoxypentose phosphates are hydrophilic. Once formed, the double-stranded DNA (or duplex DNA) forms into a helix. Helical DNA is a structure that was predicted by Watson and Crick in 1953. This DNA helix (Figure 5-4), is known as the *B form*. An A form and a Z form also occur (Wells et al, 1988) and are used by cells in special circumstances. Their structures are beyond the scope of this text, but may be seen in Mathews and van Holde (1990).

One chain of duplex DNA contains the code to synthesize specific proteins, whereas the other chain contains the template, or complement, of the code. The code itself consists of the sequence of bases in the chain. Three

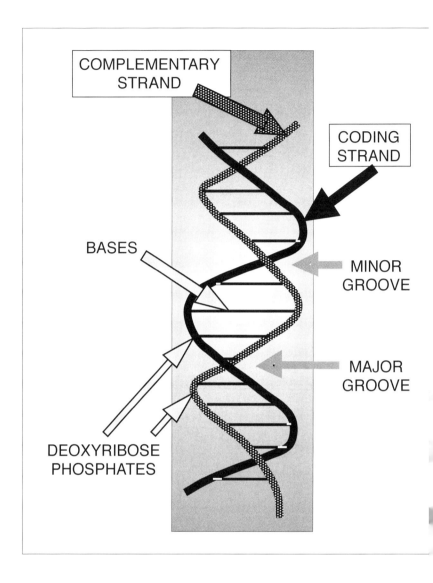

**FIGURE 5-4   A representation of the β-helical structure of duplex DNA.**
Note the presence of both a major and a minor groove in the helix. Functional proteins bind to the DNA at its major groove.

bases in succession code for a single amino acid in a protein. The genetic code is discussed in more detail later in this chapter. DNA in human cells is divided into 46 chromosomes. Each chromosome is actually a superfolded complex of proteins and duplex DNA. One chromosome contains a single, large duplex DNA molecule when the cell is not dividing. The sum of all the chromosomes in a cell constitutes the cell's *genome*. Each duplex DNA molecule contains a very large number of base pairs. The total number of base pairs in a human cell genome is about $6 \times 10^9$ (Alberts et al., 1989*a*). This is the reason that duplex DNA molecules are highly compacted and folded in the cell's nucleus. If they were not, according to Mathews and van Holde (1990) human DNA from a single cell could be strung out to a length of nearly 9 feet!

The human chromosomes typically illustrated in biology books are actually two chromosomes joined by a centromere at metaphase. A centromere is a specific DNA sequence required for cell division. Such a "chromosome" is actually two chromosomes called *chromatids* (Figure 5-5). The chromatids are composed of supercoiled structures that can be unraveled to show lengths of chromatin fibers. These fibers consist of duplex DNA wrapped around a barrellike structure of histone proteins. Strands of DNA connect each "barrel," and other nonhistone proteins are bound to the DNA at

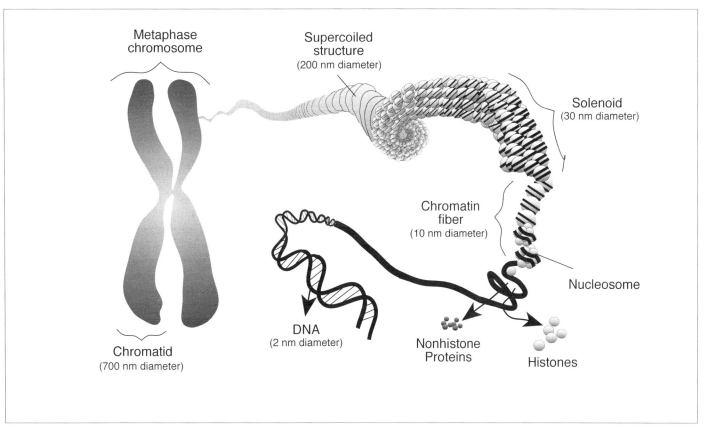

**FIGURE 5-5   Unraveling a metaphase chromosome (two DNA molecules or chromatids).**
The supercoiled structures can be untwisted to show chromatin fibers containing nucleosomes (histones and wound DNA) joined by linker DNA. The nonhistone proteins are bound to DNA between each nucleosome. (Adapted from Mathews CK, and van Holde KE. *Biochemistry.* Redwood City, CA: Benjamin/Cummings, 1990;1006.)

these strands. The histone proteins assist the DNA in compacting itself, whereas the nonhistone proteins are involved with the control of DNA and RNA processing (Figure 5-6.)

*Replication of DNA*   When a cell divides, it reproduces its DNA by a process known as *replication*. Replication is semiconservative. This means that one original strand of the "parent" duplex DNA becomes incorporated into each of the two new "daughter" duplex DNA molecules. This is to say that one coding strand and one complementary strand of each of the two new strands came from the original DNA before division.

**FIGURE 5-6   The appearance of chromatin fibers (see Figure 5-5) in greater detail.**
H1 histones appear to stabilize the DNA on the nucleosome. (Adapted from Mathews CK and van Holde KE. *Biochemistry.* Redwood City, CA: Benjamin/Cummings, 1990;1012.)

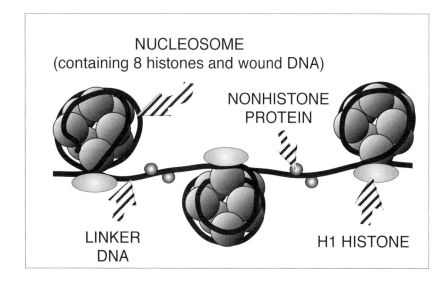

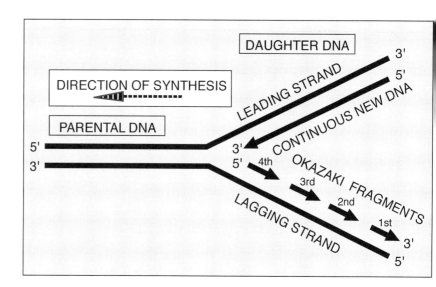

**FIGURE 5-7    Sequence scheme of daughter DNA on the leading and lagging strands.**
The numbers on the Okazaki fragments (first through fourth) indicate the order of synthesis of each fragment in time, whereas the arrows indicate their 5'→3' sequence.

Since the DNA in each chromosome is so long, replication takes place in several sites at once. It requires many proteins to carry out replication. Some of these, such as DNA polymerase, are enzymes. Each site of active replication is referred to as a *replication fork*, in which the parental DNA is the stem and each of the two daughter DNAs is a tine of the fork. Several requirements make this process complicated. For example, the helix must be unwound before replication, and synthesis of each strand must proceed from the 5' end of each added nucleotide to the 3' end of each growing strand. This may not seem complicated intuitively. However, when one realizes that each duplex DNA has its member strands oriented in opposite 5', 3' directions, a paradox becomes apparent if replication is to move in one direction. The problem is solved by the cell's genetic machinery (Figure 5-7). The figure shows a diagram of a replication fork with parental DNA on the left. In the top daughter duplex DNA the new strand is synthesized in the conventional 5'→3' direction. This strand is known as the *leading strand*. In the bottom daughter duplex DNA the new strand is made in discrete, short, discontinuous fragments (5'→3') known as *Okazaki fragments*, named for Reiji Okazaki, the scientist who discovered them (Ogawa and Okazaki, 1980). Each short fragment (although made 5'→3') is successively formed in the direction of the opening fork (the same direction as the growing, leading strand). The

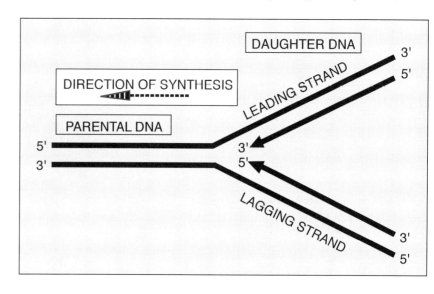

**FIGURE 5-8    The overall effective sequence of synthesis of both the leading and lagging strands.**

fragments are then joined by a ligase enzyme and become a continuous strand. In effect, the synthesis of each strand appears to be unidirectional (Figure 5-8).

The actual protein assembly of a replication fork may be seen in Figure 5-9. As can be seen in the figure, several proteins contribute to the replication process. DNA helicase, an enzyme, breaks the hydrogen bonds between the bases to form single strands. Bound to the DNA helicase is a second enzyme, RNA primase. This enzyme periodically synthesizes a short strand of primer RNA that binds to one separated parental strand. This single parental strand becomes the template for the lagging strand and the RNA primer is the initiator for the new lagging strand.

It is important that this parental strand remain a single strand at this stage. For this reason, double helix–destabilizing proteins temporarily bind to it. The parental template for the lagging strand loops around and passes through a DNA polymerase III enzyme complex, which is actually two polymerase enzymes. One enzyme (see Figure 5-9, bottom) synthesizes new DNA bound to the RNA primer to form an Okazaki fragment on the lagging strand, while the other enzyme (see Figure 5-9, top) forms the new DNA chain for the leading strand. A little farther out on the lagging strand a complex of DNA polymerase I and ligase hydrolyze the RNA primer and complete the gaps between the DNA Okazaki fragments to form a continuous strand. The ligase enzyme inserts the last nucleotide to join the fragment with the new growing strand.

## Ribonucleic Acid

Ribonucleic acid is similar chemically to DNA except for two important differences: ribose replaces deoxyribose as a pentose, and uracil (as uridine ribose monophosphate) replaces thymine as a base. Uridine 5'-monophosphate (Figure 5-10) should be compared with the bases in Figure 5-1. As a general rule, RNA is single stranded, but there are notable exceptions

**FIGURE 5-9    The actual appearance of a replication fork.**
White arrows point out the proteins involved in replication. Although similar to Figures 5-7 and 5-8, it may be seen that the parental DNA forming the lagging strand template must first loop back toward the lower DNA polymerase III molecule before an Okazaki fragment can be formed. For this reason, helix-destabilizing proteins prevent premature helical formation. (Adapted from Mathews CK, and van Holde KE. *Biochemistry.* Redwood City, CA: Benjamin/ Cummings, 1990; 850.)

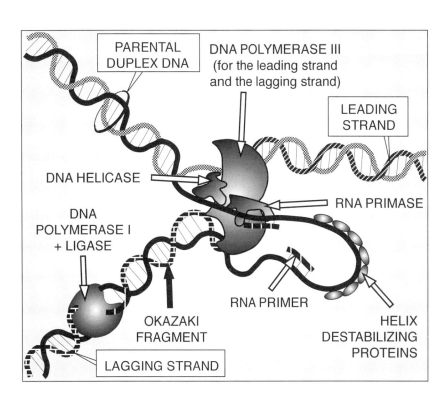

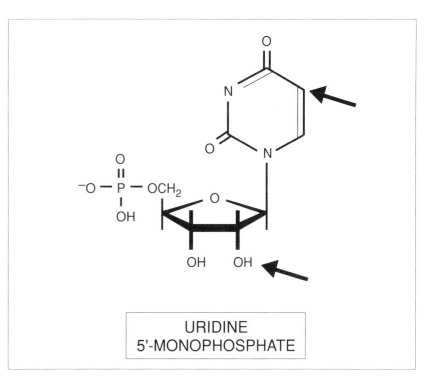

**FIGURE 5-10** Uridine 5′-monophosphate, the RNA nucleotide that is different than its corresponding DNA nucleotide (see Figure 5-1).

Uridine lacks a methyl group (*top arrow*), which is present in thymine. The ribose has a 2′ hydroxyl group (*bottom arrow*). This is the incorporated form. The precursor form is triphosphorylated.

**TABLE 5-1  Types of RNA Used in Protein Synthesis***

| Type | Approximate Size (Base Pairs) | Percentage in Cell % | Function |
|---|---|---|---|
| heterogeneous nuclear (hnRNA) | 8000 | 7 | Nuclear precursor of mRNA |
| messenger (mRNA) | 1200 | 3 | Carries the actual code for a protein |
| transfer (tRNA) | 80 | 15 | Attaches amino acids to a protein being synthesized |
| ribosomal (rRNA) | 5000, 2000, 160, 120 | 75 | Possibly catalytic for protein synthesis |

*Some hnRNA has as many as 20,000 base pairs. The mRNA size given is an average size needed to make a protein of 400 amino acids. The tRNA ranges from 70 to 90 base pairs. The rRNA consists of four types, but their role has not been shown conclusively. (See Alberts et al., [1989, p. 219].)

with some RNA-containing viruses as well as in regions of both transfer and ribosomal RNA (to be discussed).

In eukaryotic cells, the processes of producing proteins require four different kinds of RNA (Table 5-1). Heterogeneous nuclear RNA (hnRNA) is the initial coding RNA produced from DNA in the process of protein synthesis. Messenger RNA (mRNA), a cellular refinement of hnRNA made in the nucleus, is the form of RNA that carries the exact code for protein sequencing. It is interesting that mRNA represents only 3% of the total RNA present at a given time. Such a low value indicates the strict control necessary for protein synthesis. Transfer RNA (tRNA) is a short-chain RNA that attaches to specific amino acids and transports them to ribosomes, where proteins are synthesized. Ribosomal RNA (rRNA) represents 75% of all RNA in a cell and about 66% of the mass of a ribosome where it resides.

Currently, the precise role of rRNA is unknown; however, a catalytic role in protein synthesis is postulated (Lehninger et al, 1993).

*Transcription of RNA*   The synthesis of RNA from DNA is called *transcription*. In this process DNA serves as the template for new RNA formation. The RNA is made by the catalytic activity of three different RNA polymerases that are more properly called *DNA-directed RNA polymerases*. When hnRNA is formed it is the first step in protein synthesis. The polymerization is similar to DNA polymerization (replication) using nucleotide triphosphates as building blocks (see Figure 5-3). However, uridine triphosphate replaces deoxythymidine triphosphate. The three RNA polymerases are RNA polymerase I (for rRNA synthesis); RNA polymerase II (for hnRNA, and ultimately mRNA, synthesis); and RNA polymerase III (for tRNA and the smaller species of rRNA).

Transcription can begin only at a promoter site, another way of rigidly controlling protein synthesis. This site contains specific short sequences of DNA such as TATA and/or CAAT. These sequences do not code for amino acids. In addition, numerous regulatory proteins bind to this region that either support or inhibit the initiation of hnRNA synthesis. The entire region is called an *upstream promoter element*. Figure 5-11 shows such a promoter element of RNA for the eventual synthesis of β-globin proteins in chickens. These proteins bind to the DNA at their major grooves (see Figure 5-4) at linker DNA sites between nucleosomes (see Figure 5-6).

When RNA polymerase binds to the promoter element, it either proceeds downstream to begin RNA synthesis or stops depending on the combined influences of the proteins bound at the TATA, CAAT, or other promoting sequence regions. In addition, auxiliary regions of DNA called *enhancers* have further influence on hnRNA synthesis. These enhancers are discussed in Chapter 6. The operational characteristics for the control of RNA synthesis are outlined in Figure 5-12.

*The Genetic Code and Nonsense Sequences*   Previously in this chapter it was mentioned that a sequence of three bases codes for a single amino acid in a protein. A number of well-known scientists, beginning with Francis Crick

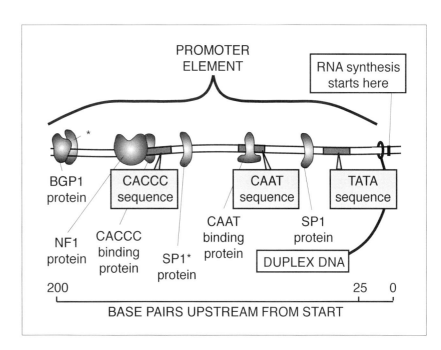

**FIGURE 5-11   An "upstream" promoter element of DNA used to control the synthesis of hnRNA for β-globin in chickens.**
Three control sequences, shown in boxes, act together along with the proteins BGP1, NF1, CACCC-binding protein, CAAT-binding protein and SP1 to turn synthesis *ON* or *OFF*. (Adapted from Alberts B, Bray D, Lewis J, Roff M, Roberts K, and Watson J. *Molecular Biology of the Cell* (2nd ed.) New York: Garland, 1989; 567.)

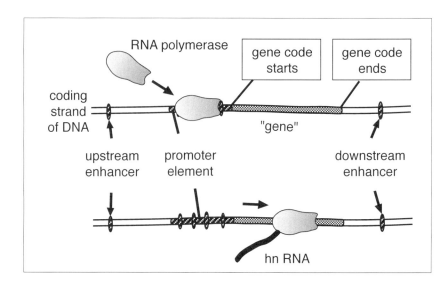

**FIGURE 5-12**   RNA polymerase must pass through the promoter element before beginning synthesis of a specific "gene" of hnRNA. If the right combination of promoter elements is not in place, synthesis cannot begin. The enhancers assist this process (see Chapter 6).

(1958), worked for nearly a decade to determine what the code is and how it works. The code is shown in Table 5-2. It is obvious that the code is redundant; that is, more than one code can signal for the same amino acid. Note that three codes signal either to begin synthesis or to incorporate an amino acid. The stop codes specify only termination of synthesis signals.

On both DNA and RNA there are *base sequences* that do not code for amino acids. Some examples on DNA are the recently mentioned sequences TATA and CAAT, which are located at promoter elements. Other highly repeated sequences such as $(ATAAACT)_n$ have rather tenuous or uncertain roles and are sometimes called *satellite DNA*. One proposed role for them is that of binding chromatids together (see Figure 5-5). In both DNA and hnRNA, gene sequences that code for either all or part of a protein are known as *exons*. Each exon is separated by a noncoding sequence known as an *intron*. Introns act as spacers and are eventually looped out of a sequence prior to protein synthesis.

**TABLE 5-2   The Genetic Code for Protein Synthesis***

| | | | |
|---|---|---|---|
| UUU Phe | UCU Ser | UAU Tyr | UGU Cys |
| UUC " | UCC " | UAC " | UGC " |
| UUA " | UCA " | UAA Stop | UGA Stop |
| UUG " | UCG " | UAG Stop | UGG Trp |
| CUU Leu | CCU Pro | CAU His | CGU Arg |
| CUC " | CCC " | CAC " | CGC " |
| CUA " | CCA " | CAA Gln | CGA " |
| CUG " | CCG " | CAG " | CGG " |
| AUU Ile | ACU Thr | AAU Asn | AGU Ser |
| AUC " | ACC " | AAC " | AGC " |
| AUA " | ACA " | AAA Lys | AGA Arg |
| AUG Met | ACG " | AAG " | AGG " |
| GUU Val | GCU Ala | GAU Asp | GGU Gly |
| GUC " | GCC " | GAC " | GGC " |
| GUA " | GCA " | GAA Gln | GGA " |
| GUG " | GCG " | GAG " | GGG " |

*This is the code for RNA (DNA uses T wherever U occurs). AUG acts as the code for both "start" and Met. UUG and GUG occasionally are start signals. UAA, UAG, and UGA code always and only for "stop."

*The Formation of mRNA*   When hnRNA is synthesized in the nucleus, it contains two or more coding genes (exons) that are separated by one or more noncoding regions (introns). In addition, hnRNA acquires a "cap" of guanosine triphosphate at its 5' end and a "tail" of 100 to 200 bases of adenosine phosphate (polyadenosine) at its 3' end. The cap has two functions: It protects the RNA from degradation and it is involved with initiation of protein synthesis. The tail may also play a role in preventing degradation. The process of mRNA formation from hnRNA is one of looping out the introns and splicing the exons together (Figure 5-13). The looping out of introns is aided by specialized small nuclear RNA. After mRNA is formed it is transported out of the nucleus.

## Protein Synthesis (Translation)

The actual formation of a *polypeptide* (a *protein* by definition if the molecular weight exceeds 10 kd) is a cooperative process between mRNA, tRNA, ribosomes, as well as other specialized proteins. Protein formation from mRNA is known as *translation*. Since mRNA has just been discussed, let us focus on tRNA. This small RNA molecule (see Table 5-1) has extensive base pair binding. A diagrammatic representation is shown in Figure 5-14 (left). The actual shape of the molecule, due to helical folding, is somewhat like that of human liver (Figure 5-14, right). The important functional regions are the *anticodon* (the three bases that match three bases [*codons*] on mRNA) and the *3' end*. The 3' end binds to a specific amino acid. In protein translation, tRNA binds to its amino acid and enters the ribosome to attach to the codon portion of mRNA, for which it is specific.

The ribosome itself is a two-part assembly with each part composed of proteins and rRNA. The smaller subunit (mass equivalent to 40 S) houses the mRNA, while the larger subunit (60 S) houses the incoming tRNAs and their amino acids. "S" stands for Svedberg unit. See the definition given in the glossary. Protein synthesis occurs when one or more ribosomes move along the mRNA chain and cause the simultaneous formation of a polypeptide. This occurs as each tRNA, with its amino acid, binds to mRNA in succession. As each amino acid comes into the 60 S subunit, it forms a peptide bond with the previous amino acid and the peptide chain lengthens

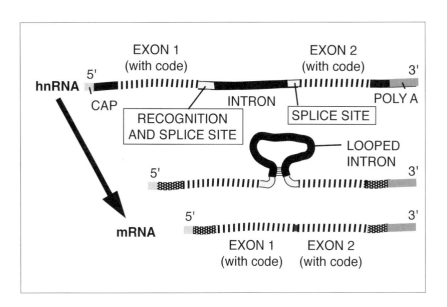

**FIGURE 5-13   The processing of hnRNA in the cell nucleus.**

Introns, noncoding spacers, are looped out of the RNA sequence by small ribonuclear protein complexes called *spliceosomes*. The remaining coded sequence is mRNA.

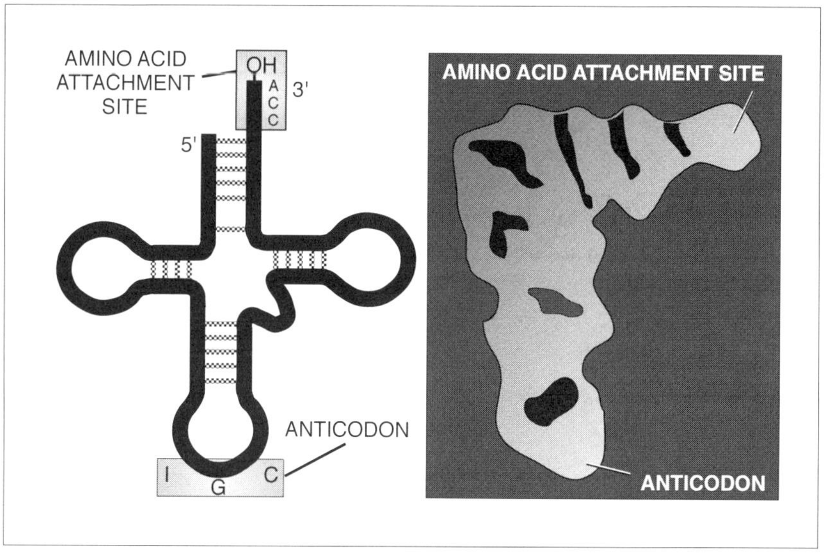

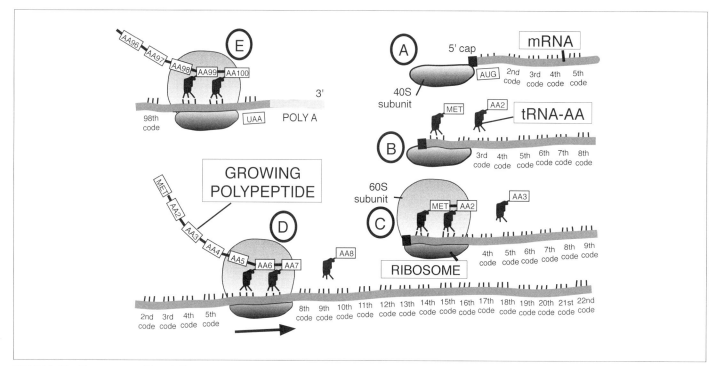

**FIGURE 5-14    Diagrams (*left*) of the tRNA for the amino acid alanine.**

The anticodon I (inosine), G (guanine), C (cytosine) matches the mRNA code GCU, GCC, or GCA (three of four codes for alanine). Inosine is one of several unusual bases found on tRNA. *Right:* diagram of the actual twisted, partially-helical shape of tRNA.

**FIGURE 5-15    The process of translation.**

Initially, at A, the 5' cap of mRNA makes contact with the 40-S subunit of a ribosome and the first codon, AUG, of mRNA signals the beginning of protein synthesis as the tRNA for methionine binds to mRNA at B in the figure. Other tRNAs bearing amino acids (AA) are nearby. At C, the 60-S subunit binds, forming a complete ribosome. Other molecules of tRNA with AAs enter the ribosome and bind to the proper codons on mRNA. As they do, a peptide bond is formed between each AA in sequence by a peptidyltransferase enzyme located in the 60-S subunit. The ribosome shifts to the next codon of mRNA, and the process continues, as one can see for the seventh AA at D. At E, the ribosome approaches the codon UAA, which will bind to releasing factors (proteins) that cause sequence termination and release of the polypeptide (in this case of 100 AAs, a protein with a molecular weight of about 12.5 kd).

by one amino acid (Figure 5-15). The ribosome moves along the mRNA as each peptide bond is formed until all of the code has been "read." Although rates vary, typically 10 proteins can be formed from one mRNA molecule in 1 minute (Alberts, 1989a). In eucaryotic cells about 12 proteins are required to cause the initiation of translation. Some ribosomes exist independently in the cytoplasm, whereas others attach themselves to the rough endoplasmic reticulum. The latter ribosomes make proteins that are used for cell membranes, lysosomes (a type of digestion compartment or "cellular stomach"), and for extracellular roles. The mechanism of protein synthesis is identical in both ocular and nonocular cells.

## Alterations of DNA and Nucleic Acid Processing

No matter what one's political or social inclinations—liberal, moderate, or traditional—all depend on the operations of nucleic acids to be very traditional and very conservative. A modification of DNA has a profound effect on an organism within which it operates. This is why DNA copies itself so faithfully and even enacts reparative mechanisms when it is damaged by outside chemical or physical forces. A practical example of how such damage may occur is the alteration of adjacent thymine or thymine-cytidine bases by ultraviolet (UV) light. This event is commonly realized in skin cells exposed to bright sunlight. UV radiation (in wavelengths near 260 nm) causes a bond to form between adjacent pyrimidines in DNA (Figure 5-16, left). These pyrimidines are located side by side in the same DNA chain rather than as base pair partners on opposite chains. As such, they are called *pyrimidine dimers*. When this reaction occurs, the DNA helix is distorted and replication cannot occur beyond the dimer. A cell having a significant amount of such damage may be doomed either to die or to mutate into a cancer cell. This is how skin cancers can develop.

Fortunately, a variety of repair mechanisms usually prevent cells from meeting such fates. One common mechanism occurs that involves the sequential activity of three enzymes: excinuclease, DNA polymerase I, and DNA ligase. The first enzyme breaks 5′, 3′ bonds approximately five to eight bases on both sides of the pyrimidine dimer. After the damaged sequence is removed, the second enzyme sequences new bases at the gap using the opposite chain as a template. The third enzyme adds the last base to join the two segments of DNA together again (Figure 5-16, right). This cut, patch, and splice mechanism operates continuously to keep DNA intact.

Sometimes, however, repair mechanisms are defective. In the rare skin disease *xeroderma pigmentosum* an inherited genetic defect makes imperfect excinuclease molecules that are unable to remove pyrimidine dimers efficiently. Persons with this disease develop skin cancer very easily, and those who do not may suffer from atrophied skin, scarred eyelids, and corneal ulcerations.

In the eye, DNA damage from UV radiation is known to initiate reparative processes also (Rapp, Jose, and Pitts, 1985). However, these are not

**FIGURE 5-16  The formation of photodamaged DNA and its repair.**
At left, a 6-4 bond between two adjacent pyrimidines on the same DNA strand, caused by UV radiation, is indicated by a dotted line. At right (A), the 6-4 photoproduct is seen to cause distortion in the duplex DNA. At B, the photoproduct plus some surrounding nucleotides are removed by breaking phosphate bonds with the enzyme: excinuclease. At C and D, DNA polymerase I replaces the missing nucleotides (5′→3′), while, at E, the enzyme ligase adds the final nucleotide to splice the broken ends of the strand.

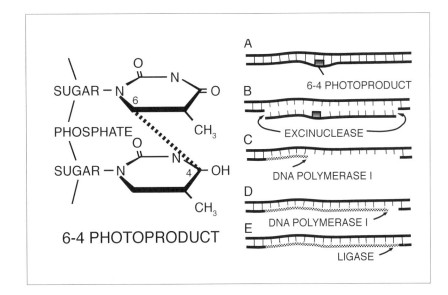

always successful, depending upon the degree, wavelength, and duration of UV exposure. Pitts et al. (1986) reported several kinds of responses in the cornea: (1) inhibition of cellular mitosis as a result of low levels of exposure; (2) swollen nuclei and cell death from moderate to high levels; and (3) complete sloughing of epithelial cells from extreme levels. At higher levels, more is involved than simple DNA damage, and the process of damage is known to be assisted by oxygen. At wavelengths shorter than 290 nm, the damage is usually confined to the corneal epithelium. At longer wavelengths the damaging effects penetrate into deeper layers of the cornea as well as the lens and the retina. Deeper penetration also requires higher-energy sources such as a mercury-xenon lamp to produce DNA damage (Pitts, 1986). Of course, UV radiation is also suspect in producing cataracts (see Chapter 1, Cataract Formation).

In addition to UV radiation (which excites electrons to produce the kind of reactions seen with DNA damage), *x-rays* and *γ-rays* are known to produce even greater damage because they possess a higher content of electromagnetic radiation and displace even those electrons that are closest to the nuclei of atoms (Daniels and Alberty, 1961). This often affects the bases in DNA. A number of chemical substances can also damage DNA. Among the most well-known chemicals are alkylating agents, chemicals that form covalent alkyl bridges between guanine, adenine, thymine, or cytosine bases on different chains of duplex DNA. Some examples are chlorambucil, carmustine, and busulfan (Figure 5-17). Ironically, these agents are used to treat cancer. That is, they are used to damage the DNA in cancerous cells so that they cannot reproduce (Korolkovas and Burckhalter. 1976).

Some chemicals are extremely dangerous. Two-naphthylamine (see Figure 5-17), which was commonly used in the chemical industry at one time, was known to cause bladder cancer in every exposed worker at one British factory where the substance was being produced (Alberts et al., 1989a). Although the list of such chemicals is continuously growing, the damaging effects of some substances are probably overstated due to the presence of

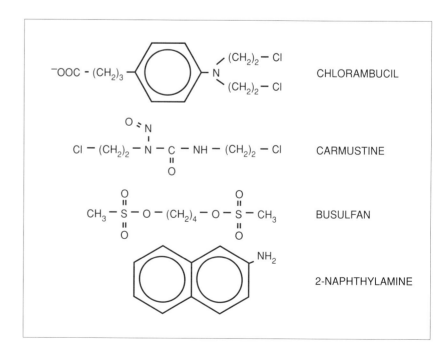

**FIGURE 5-17   DNA-modifying chemicals.**
The top three are alkylating agents that add hydrocarbon bridges (principally methylene —CH$_2$— groups) between bases on opposite sides of DNA strands. These agents are used to modify (i.e., kill) carcinoma cells. Two-naphthylamine, on the bottom, modifies the DNA of bladder cells so that they lose control of cell division (i.e., become carcinogenic).

the previously mentioned repair mechanisms. It is also important to understand that exposure to such agents, even those that are considered dangerous, must be chronic (continuous over a period of time) in order to induce a tumor growth. A single mutation of DNA is insufficient to cause cancer, and those that develop from external agents often do so only after many years of delay (Alberts et al., 1989b).

Mutations that eventually lead to cancer are disastrous, since they cause cells to lose control of their ability to divide. One or more genes within such cells modified by base alterations can then make excessive amounts of proteins that signal the cells to divide continuously or cause inactivation of genes that suppress division. These are proteins that bind to DNA promoter regions. One can consider, for example, the rare childhood ocular disease: retinoblastoma. In its hereditary form retinoblastoma consists in the uncontrolled growth that is initiated by neural precursor cells in the immature retina. There may be multiple tumors (masses of abnormal cells) present in both eyes before the end of the 3rd year of life (Vaughan and Asbury, 1980). In this case, an Rb1 gene on chromosome 13 is absent or nonfunctional. This gene, which makes proteins that suppress cell division, is one of a pair, of such genes and its absence is sufficient to allow occasional uncontrolled division to take place from failure of the other gene. It would normally make proteins of the type found in Figure 5-11. This disease is shown in Figure 5-18.

## Molecular Biology of Crystallins

Crystallins are the major soluble proteins in lens cells. As discussed in Chapter 1, much interest and study has been invested in this protein class because of its role in supporting lens development, lens clarity, and its association with the development of senile cataracts. For each major crystallin type in vertebrates it is known that there are two genes with three exons per gene for α-crystallins, six genes with six exons per gene for β-crystallins, and seven genes with three exons per gene for γ-crystallins (Piatigorsky, 1989). This amounts to 63 separate DNA and RNA sequences

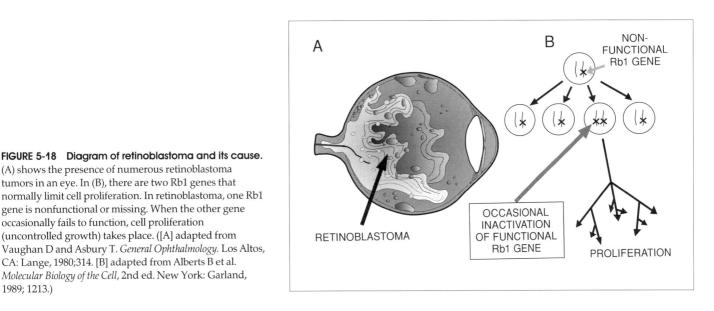

**FIGURE 5-18   Diagram of retinoblastoma and its cause.** (A) shows the presence of numerous retinoblastoma tumors in an eye. In (B), there are two Rb1 genes that normally limit cell proliferation. In retinoblastoma, one Rb1 gene is nonfunctional or missing. When the other gene occasionally fails to function, cell proliferation (uncontrolled growth) takes place. ([A] adapted from Vaughan D and Asbury T. *General Ophthalmology*. Los Altos, CA: Lange, 1980;314. [B] adapted from Alberts B et al. *Molecular Biology of the Cell*, 2nd ed. New York: Garland, 1989; 1213.)

that may be used to make only three major protein types in the human lens. The genes that determine the synthesis of α-crystallins are located on separate chromosomes. That is to say, that they are unlinked. This is partially true for the genes of the β-crystallins and not true at all for the γ-crystallin genes. One of the most amazing facts about crystallins is their diversity of types. Although three types (and many subtypes) occur in humans there are currently some 13 types known in the animal kingdom (Piatigorsky and Wistow, 1991).

On an evolutionary basis, all crystallins appear to be related to proteins that were originally made for another (nonocular) purpose before their adaptive use in the ocular lens. It is known that the α-crystallins, for example, are related to heat shock proteins. The latter are proteins which are made in response to an unusual temperature rise in an organism. They protect the organism by solubilizing and refolding any heat-denatured proteins (Alberts et al., 1989c). This is the chaperone function discussed in Chapter 1. The human crystallins have developed, apparently, by duplication of genes that made (or make) proteins in other species for a different role. It is also apparent that a variety of proteins could fulfill the requirements of a structurally clear protein to inhabit the interior of lens fiber cells. One reason, therefore, that gene studies are being pursued is that a common feature present in all the crystallin genes that distinguishes them as lens proteins might be found.

An important requirement of lens proteins is that they be synthesized in large quantities. When one considers that the genetic machinery of lens fiber cells shuts down as the cells mature, it becomes crucial for the young cell to produce very many proteins. Interest in this area dates back to the turn of the century, when biologists attempted to determine why a lens would develop from a detached epithelial tissue mass (or lens vesicle) adjacent to the fetal eye cup (developing retina). One hypothesis has been that increasing the volume of the developing primary fiber cells has the effect of causing lens formation (Figure 5-19). This is to say that the relatively rapid synthesis of crystallins during lens fiber cell differentiation promotes the elongation of that cell type by filling it with proteins. Whatever factors turn

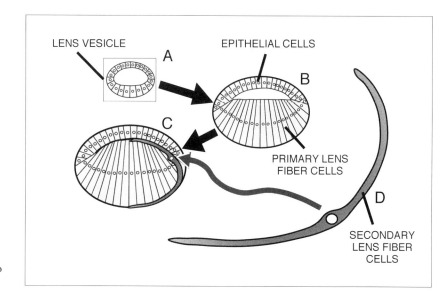

**FIGURE 5-19   Development of the lens.**
The developing fetal lens, which begins as an epithelial vesicle at A, is stimulated by both intralenticular and extralenticular factors to increase in size posteriorly at first. This is seen by the lengthening of primary lens fiber cells (A, B, C). Then the lens continues to grow by the development of secondary lens fiber cells (D). The accelerated production of crystallin proteins in these cells contributes to the volume increase (lengthening) of these cells.

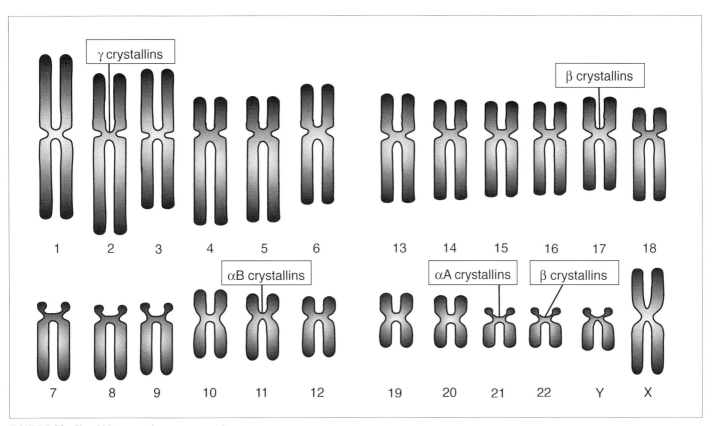

**FIGURE 5-20    The 46 human chromosomes at metaphase (double sets of chromosomes 1 through 22 as well as X and Y).**
The synthesis of lens crystallins originates at chromosomes 2, 11, 17, 21, and 22.

on the crystallin-producing genes has not yet to be accurately determined. It has been known for some time that some of these factors originate from the eye cup.

Here a gene is defined as a DNA sequence that determines a distinct polypeptide chain or code for a member of a set of closely related polypeptides (protein isoforms). See Alberts et al. (1989c) for further discussion. The locations of most of the human crystallin genes are known. The αA-crystallin genes occur on chromosome 21 (Quax-Jenken et al., 1985), whereas αB-crystallin genes are found on chromosome 11 (Ngo et al., 1989). Two of the eight β-crystallin genes are found on chromosomes 17 and 22, whereas all six γ-crystallin genes occur on chromosome 2 (Figure 5-20). The length and sequence of crystallin genes and their promoter sequences have been extensively investigated in recent years. For example, the mouse αA-crystallin gene and its promoter are shown in Figure 5-21. In the promoter element of that gene, only the TATA sequence has been found. There are no CACC or CAAT sequences (see Figure 5-11).

A nuclear protein termed αA-*CRYBP1* has been discovered that binds to the promoter at sequences $-66$ to $-57$ (Nakamura et al., 1990). This protein contains so-called zinc fingers, which help the protein to bind to the aforementioned DNA sequences at their major grooves (Figure 5-22). Slight conformational differences in promoter DNA sequences and the shape of the protein zinc fingers determine where the protein will bind to the DNA. In the case of protein αA-CRYBP1, Nakamura et al. suggest that its binding is necessary for the normal initiation of αA-crystallin synthesis. That is, it is necessary for the synthesis (transcription) of hnRNA, which codes for this crystallin. This control is separate from the extralenticular gene controls, which will be considered in Chapter 6.

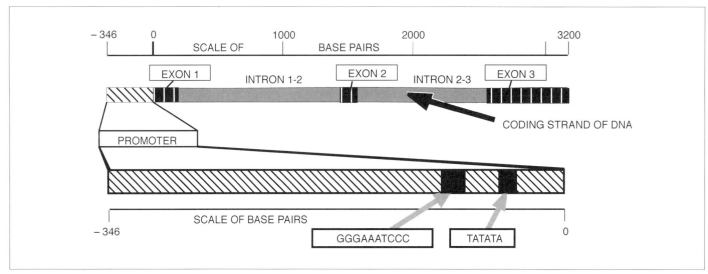

**FIGURE 5-21  The region of DNA that codes for mouse αA-crystallin with its promoter.**
It has three exons separated by two introns. The promoter region (magnified) has a sequence (GGGAAATCCC) that binds to a protein called αA-CRYBPI, which is necessary for transcription. (Adapted from Nakamura T et al, 1990.)

It should be apparent from the preceding discussion that any chemical or physical process that produces a defective gene, transmits (by replication) a defective gene, or either turns on or shuts down any gene necessary for normal cell function will result in some pathological process or disease. This is just as true for the eye as for any other part of the body. Defective genes that may be involved in hereditary cataract formation, for example, have been studied in animal models that have defects similar to those in humans. This study is important inasmuch as human congenital cataracts are relatively common. However, a large variety of congenital cataract types exist and a limited line of traceable descent makes it difficult to classify them in each individual. Zigler (1990) has described six animal models with traceable pedigrees and congenital cataract types that may be useful. In one of these, the Philly mouse, it was found that the cataract that began to form 15 days after birth was due to a deficiency of a β-crystallin (Carper et al., 1982). Subsequently, it was shown that the β-crystallin, a βB2 subtype, is not made due to the mutation of its gene. Instead, the gene makes a defective substitute protein (Nakamura et al., 1988). According to Zigler, cataract formation in the Frazer mouse and in 13/N guinea pigs can also be traced to abnormal genes that make defective crystallins. In humans, attempts to locate the genes responsible for congenital cataracts have only recently begun.

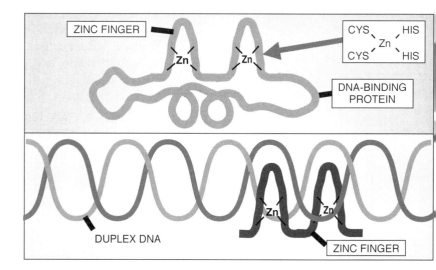

**FIGURE 5-22  Zinc finger attachment to DNA.**
Proteins binding to DNA have zinc fingers, regions that slip into the major grooves of DNA. Zinc binds to four amino acids (two CYS and two HIS) on the peptide chain to form the finger shape. (Adapted from Alberts B et al. *Molecular Biology of the Cell*, 2nd ed. New York: Garland, 1989; 490.)

## Viral Intervention in the Cornea

Viruses are relatively simple organisms compared to eucaryotes. They depend on higher organisms to carry out their reproduction. This is accomplished by using the genetic machinery of host cells. Although it is simplistic to say that a virus is itself a bag of genes, such a description is fairly accurate. Viruses exist in a variety of shapes, sizes, and complexities. The more simple ones have only an outside coat or bag known as a *capsid* composed of several types of proteins. The capsid, in more complex viruses, may be covered by a lipid membrane obtained from viral hosts. The lipid membrane also contains proteins. Either DNA or RNA is found within the capsid. Viral nucleic acids may be either single- or double-stranded with some variations in the shape of the strands. Table 5-3 lists some of the commonly known viruses.

In the cornea, one of the more serious viral infections is initiated by herpes viruses, especially herpes simplex (types 1 and 2). This virus contains double-stranded DNA (Table 5-3), and its capsid is covered by both a granular zone and a membrane envelope (Figure 5-23). Herpes simplex is a pervasive virus. In the United States, 90% of the population becomes infected with type 1 by the time they are 15 years of age (Burns, 1963), though only a small (but significant) fraction of this percentage develop corneal infections.

The herpes simplex virus is capable of existing in two states. In one state it actively infects cells and reproduces. In the other state, it becomes quiescent in its host for prolonged periods of time. The mechanisms for attachment/invasion, reproduction, and egress from the infected cell are shown in Figure 5-24. The virus particle (virion) attaches itself to the cell membrane or corneal epithelial cells by binding to a proteoglycan (Roizman and Sears, 1991) associated with the membrane surface (the glycocalyx mentioned in Chapter 4 under Cell Membranes). The viral envelope fuses to the cell membrane, and the capsid, with its duplex DNA, is taken rapidly into the cell. The capsid is transported to the nuclear pores of the cells, where viral DNA is released into the nucleus. There, viral transcription occurs to produce viral mRNA, which is diffused to the cell's cytoplasm, where three different classes of viral proteins are made in sequence: regulatory or $\alpha$-proteins, viral DNA replication or $\beta$-proteins, and capsid structural or $\gamma$-proteins. The virus requires a high concentration of $\beta$-proteins, including its own viral DNA polymerase, to replicate its own viral DNA, which is the next step. The capsids are assembled from viral $\gamma$-proteins in the nucleus by

**TABLE 5-3    Characteristics of Some Viruses**

| Virus | Nucleic Acid/Form/Length* | Capsid[†] | Activity Causes |
|---|---|---|---|
| Poliovirus | RNA/single-stranded/7440 b | Simple | Paralytic poliomyelitis |
| Reoviris | RNA/double-stranded/1196-3896 bp | Simple | Colorado tick fever |
| Parvovirus | DNA/single-stranded/4680-5176 b | Simple | Animal infections |
| Bacteriophage[‡] | DNA/single-stranded, circular/5700 b | Simple | Infections in bacteria |
| Herpesvirus | DNA/double-stranded/150,000 bp | Projections | Epithelial and ocular infections |
| Polyoma | DNA/double-stranded, circular/5000 bp | Simple | Demyelinating disease |
| Adenovirus | DNA/duplex, linked protein/35,937 bp | Projections | Respiratory and ocular disease |
| Poxvirus | DNA/duplex, sealed ends/to 300,000 bp | Covered | Smallpox and ocular infections |

*Key: b, bases; bp, base pairs; duplex, double-stranded.

[†]Capsids are geometrical proteins. Some are uncovered (simple); some have membrane covers (covered) and/or protein projections (projections).

[‡]$\phi\chi$174

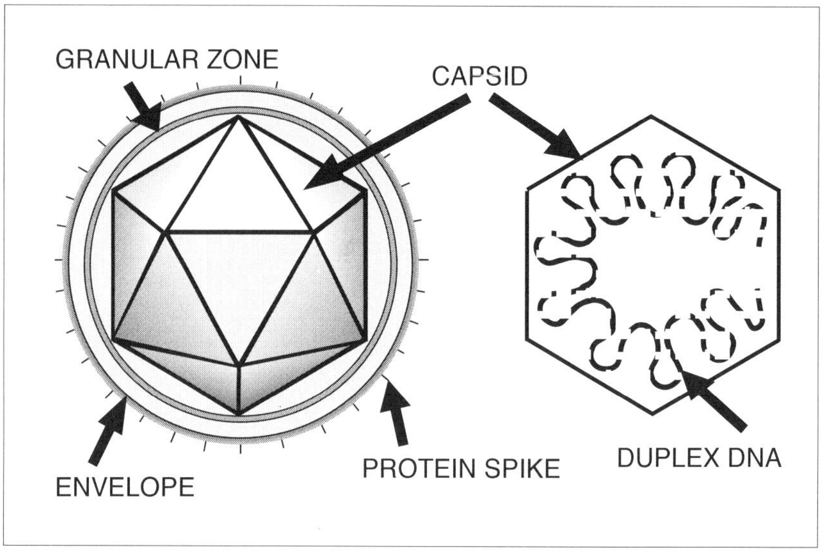

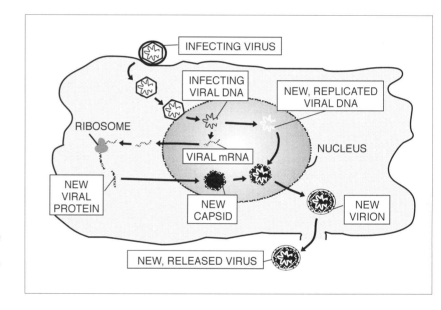

**FIGURE 5-23** Diagram of a herpes virus unit, or virion. At left, the capsid is surrounded by a granular zone, or tegument, of protein, which is covered by an envelope of membrane. Projecting from the membrane are protein spikes. Within the capsid (an icosahedron = 20 sides), as shown on the right, a single length of duplex DNA is packed in the form of a toroid. (Adapted from Roizman B, Whitley RJ, and Lopez C, eds. *The Human Herpesviruses.* New York: Raven Press, 1993:2 and 29.)

**FIGURE 5-24** Diagram of herpes virus infecting a cell. After making contact and binding to the host cell, the capsid is internalized and binds to the nuclear membrane. Viral DNA is released into the membrane, where it replicates and transcribes itself. New viral proteins are made from the mRNA on host ribosomes. At the third stage of translation capsid proteins form new capsids in the nucleus. DNA enters the capsids, and the virion acquires its membrane from the nucleus. The virion leaves the cell by reverse phagocytosis.

a process that has not yet been defined. Afterward, newly replicated viral DNA is packaged in the capsids (see Figure 5-23). The completed virion passes through the nuclear membrane, where it becomes coated or enveloped with nuclear membrane and eventually is ejected from the cell by a mechanism akin to reversed phagocytosis. The virion is ready, at this point, to infect another cell.

What is destructive or pathological about this process is that those cells which are used by the virus are eventually killed. This occurs for three reasons: destruction of the host nucleolus (where ribosomes are made), terminal alteration of host membranes (especially at the nucleus), and shutdown of host protein synthesis. In the cornea, such a destructive process can be visualized as dendritic (branchlike) ulcers in which the virus has killed epithelial cells (Figure 5-25).

A final but significant property of herpes viral infections is the phenomenon of *latency*. After a primary infection, virus particles are transported by sensory nerves to automatic ganglia. In the case of a corneal infection, the virus particles become stored in the cells of the gasserian ganglion (on the

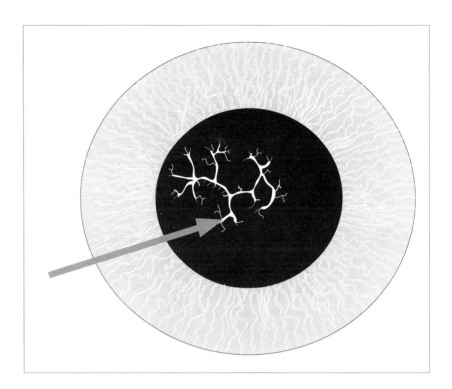

**FIGURE 5-25    A cornea, with its posterior surrounding iris, infected by herpes virus (*gray arrow*).**
The diagram shows the typical dendritic lesions of cells killed by this virus.

larger root of the fifth cranial nerve) and they remain inactive there until they are reactivated by some stressful stimulus such as emotional trauma, fever, sunburn, or menstruation. Then the viral particles travel back to the cornea and reinfect it. The mechanisms of the formation of latency and viral reactivation are currently not understood. It is known that in latency the viral DNA becomes circular and produces one hnRNA known as LAT1 (latency-associated transcript) RNA (Roizman and Sears, 1991). Perhaps the products of this RNA prevent further transcription.

Clinically, herpes virus infections can be treated and controlled by several drugs that act as nucleoside analogues. For example, acycloguanosine resembles deoxyguanosine but has no pentose (Figure 5-26). Acycloguanosine is catalyzed by viral thymidine kinase in infected cells to acycloguanosine triphosphate (AGT). However, cellular thymidine kinase will not

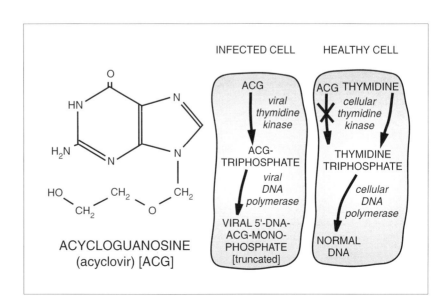

**FIGURE 5-26    Acycloguanosine and its effects on viral infected cells.**
Acycloguanosine (*left*) is a base analogue of guanosine without a pentose. It is an unusual substrate for viral thymidine kinase. In infected cells, ACG-triphosphate is incorporated into new viral DNA and halts (truncates) replication. Healthy cells are not affected.

phosphorylate it. Viral DNA polymerase incorporates AGT into newly formed viral DNA, as though it were deoxyguanosine triphosphate. This immediately halts further replication, since the polymerase cannot link new bases past the acycloguanosine. This is due to the lack of a 3' hydroxy group on the molecule (Elion, 1983). In effect, the infection is halted. Since uninfected cells do not catalyze acycloguanosine, the drug is nontoxic to healthy cells. If the herpes virus were not able to enter a latent stage, corneal herpes could be completely cured.

## Summary

Nucleic acids exist in two forms, DNA and RNA. DNA preserves the cellular genome while RNA translates the code of the genome into proteins. The process of DNA synthesis is called *replication*, whereas that of RNA synthesis is called *transcription*. When RNA produces proteins, by a process known as *translation*, four kinds of RNA are involved: heterogeneous nuclear, messenger, transfer, and ribosomal RNA. The genetic code consists of specific three base sequences for each amino acid plus some START and STOP sequences.

Protein synthesis involves the formation of peptides at ribosomes as the code sequence of mRNA is passed through each ribosome. A peptide bond is formed between each amino acid as it is brought to the ribosome by tRNA. This process is identical in all ocular and nonocular tissues. Damage to DNA in all cells can occur from UV radiation as well as from some types of chemicals. Such damage may cause cell death or uncontrolled cell division. However, reparative processes can fix many kinds of DNA damage.

In the eye, extensive investigations have shown the genetic location and some control mechanisms for the synthesis of different kinds of lens crystallins. The high synthetic rate of lens crystallins can explain how lens development takes place in embryos. Although complete information is lacking, the formation of defective crystallins in hereditary animal models of cataract formation has directed efforts to the investigation of human hereditary cataracts.

Viruses are relatively simple organisms consisting, essentially, of a protein capsid containing nucleic acids in one of several forms. Viruses enter cells and take charge of their genetic machinery to reproduce themselves. One example, herpes virus, may invade corneal cells and reproduce itself on the corneal surface. Unfortunately, herpes and other viruses usually destroy the cells which they infect. In the case of herpes viruses, the virions may enter a dormant stage (latency) in nerve ganglia and then become reactivated after a traumatic stimulus. The replication of herpes DNA may be prevented by using base analogues that become incorporated into the viral DNA and prevent further synthesis.

## References

Alberts B, Bray D, Lewis J, Raff M, Roberts K, and Watson J. *In Molecular Biology of the Cell*, 2nd ed. New York: Garland, 1989a;1187–1218.

Alberts B, Bray D, Lewis J, Raff M, Roberts K, and Watson J. *In Molecular Biology of the Cell*, 2nd ed. New York: Garland, 1989b;420–421.

Alberts B, Bray D, Lewis J, Raff M, Roberts K, and Watson J. *In Molecular Biology of the Cell*, 2nd ed. New York: Garland, 1989c;591–592.

Beebe D. Growth factors in the eye. *In* Piatigorsky J, Shinohara T, and Zelenka PS (eds.) *Molecular Biology of the Eye.* New York: Liss, 1988;457–460.

Burns, RP. A double-blind study of IDU in human herpes simplex keratitis. *Arch Ophthalmol* 1963;70:381–384.

Carper D, Shinohara T, Piatigorsky J, and Kinoshita KJH. Deficiency of functional messenger RNA for a developmentally regulated β-crystallin polypeptide in a hereditary cataract. *Science* 1982;217:463–464.

Crick FHC. On protein synthesis. *Symp Soc Exp Biol* 1958;12:138–162.

Daniels F, and Alberty RA. *Physical Chemistry,* 2nd ed. New York: John Wiley & Sons, 1961;517–518.

Elion GB. The biochemistry and mechanism of action of acyclovir. *J Antimicrob Chemother* 1983;12(Suppl B):9–17.

Korolkovas A, and Burckhalter JH. Essentials of Medicinal Chemistry. *New York: John Wiley & Sons,* 1976; 541–546.

Lehninger AL, Nelson DL, and Cox MM. *Principles of Biochemistry,* 2nd ed. New York: Worth, 1993:887.

Mathews CK, and van Holde KE. *Biochemistry.* Redwood City, CA: Benjamin/Cummings, 1990;105–108, 1001–1004.

Nakamura M, Russell P, Carper DA, Inana G, and Kinoshita, JH. Alteration of a developmentally regulated, heat-stable polypeptide in the lens of the Philly mouse. *J Biol Chem* 1988;263:19218–19221.

Nakamura T, Donovan DM, Hamada K, Sax CM, Norman B, Flanagan JR, Ozato K, Westphal H, and Piatigorsky J. Regulation of the mouse αA-crystallin gene: isolation of a cDNA encoding a protein that binds to a cis sequence motif shared with the major histocompatibility complex class I gene and other genes. *Molecular Cell Biol* 1990;10:3700–3708.

Ngo JT, Klisak I, Dubin RA, Piatigorsky J, Mohandos T, Sparkes RS, and Bateman JB. Assignment of the α-B-crystallin gene to human chromosome 11. *Genomics* 1989;5:665-669.

Ogawa T, and Okazaki T. Discontinuous DNA replication. *Annu Rev Biochem* 1980;49:421–457.

Piatigorsky J. Lens crystallins and their genes: Diversity and tissue-specific expression. *FASEB* J 1989;3:1933–1940.

Piatigorsky J, and Wistow G. The recruitment of crystallins: New functions precede gene duplication. *Science* 1991;252:1078–1079.

Pitts D. A position paper on ultraviolet radiation. *In* Cronly-Dillon J, Rosen ES, and Marshall J (eds). *Hazards of Light.* New York: Pergamon Press, 1986;209–219.

Pitts DG, Chu LWF, Bergmanson JPG, and Jose JG. Damage and recovery in the UV exposed cornea. *In* Cronly-Dillon J, Rosen ES, Marshall J (eds). *Hazards of Light.* New York: Pergamon Press, 1986;209–219.

Quax-Jenken Y, Quax W, van Reus G, Khan PM, and Bloemendal H. Complete structure of the αB crystallin gene: Conservation of the exon-intron distribution in the two non-linked alpha crystallin genes. *Proc Natl Acad Sci USA* 1985;82:5819–5823.

Rapp LM, Jose JG, and Pitts DG. DNA repair synthesis in the rat retina following in vivo exposure to 300 nm radiation. *Invest Ophthalmol Vis Sci* 1985;26:384–388.

Roizman B, and Sears AE. Herpes simplex viruses and their replication. In Fields BN, and Knipe DM (eds). *Fundamental Virology*, 2nd ed. New York Raven Press, 1991;878–882.

Vaughan D, and Asbury T. *General Ophthalmology*. Los Altos, CA: Lange Medical, 1980;314.

Watson JD, and Crick FHC. Molecular structure of nucleic acids. *Nature* 1953;171:737–738.

Wells, R, Collier DA, Hanvey JC, Shimizu M, and Wohlrab F. The chemistry and biology of unusual DNA structures adopted by oligopurine-oligopyrimidine sequences. *FASEB* J 1988;2:2939–2949.

Zigler, JA. Animal models for the study of maturity-onset and hereditary cataract. *Exp Eye Res* 1990; 50:651–657.

# Chapter 6

# Hormones

## Functions and Types

The complexity of multi-cellular organisms, including humankind, requires the use of biochemical mechanisms that will maintain control and cooperation among all the member cells of that organism. Some biochemical control mechanisms have already been presented in the discussion of enzyme regulation of metabolic pathways (Chapters 2 and 3). However, such regulations are confined within individual cells. Here we deal with the regulation of *intercellular* processes such as glucose uptake into cells, sexual maturation, physiological drive and mood, and blood flow, among others.

The hypothalamus, along with certain organs (endocrine glands), release chemical messengers to direct specific classes of cells to alter their functions. These messengers are called: *hormones* (from the Greek *horman*, to set into motion). Hormones now also include chemical messengers that function entirely within a cell. That is, they deliver biochemical messages from one part of a cell to another. In the eye, intercellular hormones do not directly affect vision, but help to maintain it at an unaltered, high-quality level. Moreover, a cellular internal hormone mechanism is directly activated by light to bring about visual transduction, as though light itself were acting as a hormone. Certain forms of hormonal pathology, unfortunately, can affect the eye as an organ and, eventually, bring about a loss of visual quality.

Hormones are released into the bloodstream to certain "targeted" cells. These are cells that either have receptors (proteins) for the hormone at their plasma membrane surface or are capable of binding the hormone at specific locations on their DNA in the nucleus. Cells also have internal hormones called *second messengers* that are activated by those exterior hormones that bind to the cell surface. The second messenger operates within the cell at a variety of intracellular targets (e.g., cell membranes, Golgi apparatus, nucleus) and brings about one or more physiological responses. Those hormones that enter a cell bind to an intracellular receptor protein and then migrate and bind to a DNA enhancer (Chapter 5). After binding to the enhancer, the hormone causes an increase or decrease in protein synthesis, which also results in one or more physiological responses. The mechanisms of these two extracellular hormone types are shown in Figure 6-1.

A given class of cells may also affect its close neighbor cells by secreting local hormones. These hormones affect only a small surrounding area, and this is referred to as a *paracrine function*. When local hormones affect the same cells that produce them, the term *autocrine hormone* is sometimes used. In effect, therefore, it is possible to distinguish four hormone classes: endocrine hormones that bind to a cellular surface, endocrine hormones that enter a cell and bind to its DNA, intracellular hormones (second messengers), and paracrine hormones, whose effects are only local.

In the endocrine system, there exist primary, secondary, and tertiary targeted cells. Initially hormone release originates from cells of the hypothalamus (hypothalamic nuclei) to targeted cells of the anterior pituitary gland, the primary target tissue, by way of the portal vein (Figure 6-2). These hormones are often called *releasing factors*. The hypothalamus itself

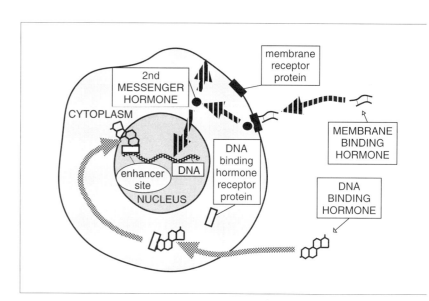

**FIGURE 6-1    General scheme of hormone interaction with a cell.**

Membrane-binding hormones (from endocrine and paracrine cells) bind to a membrane receptor protein on the cell surface. This activates (or deactivates) the formation of a second messenger within the cell hormone. The second messenger hormone causes amplified biochemical reactions in the cell. DNA-binding hormones (from endocrine cells only) penetrate the cell and bind to a cytoplasmic DNA-binding hormone receptor protein. The hormone-protein complex diffuses to the nucleus, where it binds to an enhancer site on DNA. Such binding affects the synthesis (or nonsynthesis) of specific proteins in the cell.

**FIGURE 6-2    General scheme of the endocrine system of hormones.**

Initiation of hormone release most often begins in the hypothalamus, where there are two systems to activate the release of hormones from the anterior and posterior pituitary. Hypothalamic cells release hormones into the portal blood vessel, where they are carried to cells of the anterior pituitary. Paraventricular and supraoptic cells synapse directly with cells of the posterior pituitary. They communicate with them by the release of neurotransmitters (see Chapter 7). Cells of the pituitary are primary target cells of the endocrine system. The primary target cells release a variety of hormones (peptides), including thyroid-stimulating hormone (TSH), growth hormone (GH), luteinizing hormone (LH), oxytocin (OT), and vasopressin (VP) to secondary cells. The notable exceptions to this system are the cells of the adrenal medulla, which are targeted by neurotransmitters from the sympathetic nervous system (see Chapter 7), and, for the most part, the cells of the pancreas (although growth hormone also influences those cells). The pancreas usually reacts to levels of blood glucose and other nutrients in a somewhat autonomous fashion. Secondary targeted cells, receiving input from the anterior pituitary, release hormones to a wide variety of tertiary targeted cells (only a limited number are shown here). The hormones (amino acid derivatives, peptides, and steroids) include: $T_3$ and $T_4$ (triiodothyronine and thyroxine), CORT (cortisone), EPI (epinephrine), insulin, estradiol, and testosterone. The eyes are a tertiary target tissue also. "Other tissues*" represents every other cell type.

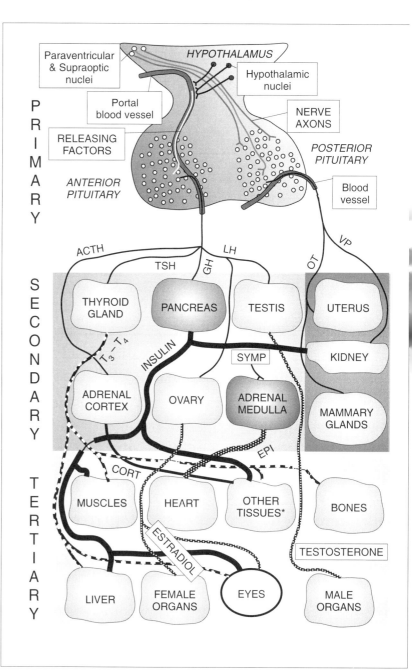

**TABLE 6-1    Peptide, Protein and Amino Acid Derived Hormones***

| Hormone | Molecular Weight | Source | Target | Mechanism | Effect |
|---|---|---|---|---|---|
| Thyrotropin-releasing hormone[†] | 363 | Hypothalamus | Anterior pituitary | Membrane receptor/ second messenger | Releases thyrotropin |
| Growth hormone | 22,000 | Anterior pituitary | Pancreas | Membrane receptor/ second messenger | Releases insulin and growth factors |
| Corticotropin | 4500 | Anterior pituitary | Adrenal cortex | Membrane receptor/ second messenger | Releases adrenal steroids |
| Thyrotropin | 26,600 | Anterior pituitary | Thyroid gland | Membrane receptor/ second messenger | Releases $T_3$ and $T_4$ |
| Oxytocin | 1007 | Posterior pituitary | Uterus; breasts | Membrane receptor/ second messenger | Contraction; milk release |
| Vasopressin | 1084 | Posterior pituitary | Kidney; muscles[‡] | Membrane receptor/ second messenger | Resorption of Na/water |
| Insulin | 6000 | Pancreas | Liver, other | Membrane receptor/ second messenger | Glucose and amino acid uptake |
| Glucagon | 3485 | Pancreas | Liver, other | Membrane receptor/ second messenger | Release of glucose, ketones |
| Thyroxine ($T_4$)[§] | 777 | Thyroid gland | Liver, other | DNA enhancer | Stimulation of metabolism |

*This list is selective. The reader should consult with other texts for other hormones in this classification.

†There are separate releasing/inhibitory hormones for each of the anterior pituitary hormones.

‡Smooth muscles only.

§Four iodine groups.

causes hormone release in response to a variety of stimuli that reach the brain—cold, heat, trauma, hunger, satiety, and fear among them. Certain cells (paraventricular and supraoptic nuclei) of the hypothalamus also make direct synaptic connection to cells of the posterior pituitary gland, such that a nerve depolarization to these cells is equivalent to the primary hormone release to cells of the anterior pituitary.

Stimulation of pituitary cells, anterior and posterior, by primary hormones or nervous discharge causes the release of other hormones to secondary target tissues (e.g., thyroid gland, ovary, adrenals). Most of the secondary tissue cells then release their own hormones to tertiary target tissues (e.g., muscles, bones, liver). At this stage, the hormones elicit those cell responses that can bring about a physiological response due to altered enzyme activity and either increased, decreased, or otewise modified protein production. This "pecking order" of cell targeting has the advantage of both amplifying the physiological effects required as well as producing the effects in a controlled, coordinated manner. Such effects can range from very short periods of time (prostaglandins act for only seconds) to extended periods (growth hormone can have effects that last for days). On average, however, the effects are usually short lived. Part of the reason for this is that the hormones themselves have a short existence prior to their enzymatic degradation. Prostaglandins, for example, usually fail to survive a single pass through the circulatory system (Mathews & van Holde, 1990). In addition, the hormones that are released are present in very small quantities ($10^{-9}$ to $10^{-12}$ M).

Hormones fall into five biochemical classes: peptides or proteins, amino acid derivatives, steroids, cyclic nucleotides, and eicosanoids. Representative peptides and proteins, as well as amino acid derivatives, are given in Table 6-1 with their mechanism of action, biochemical, and physiological

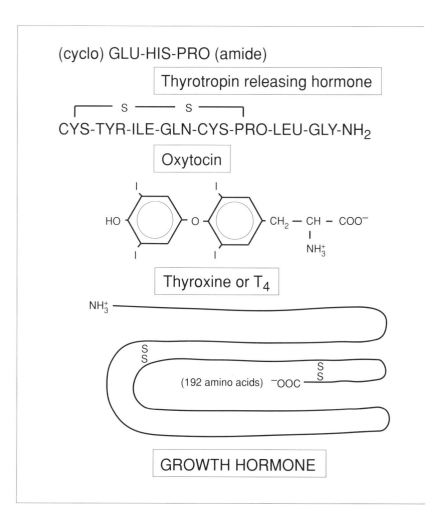

FIGURE 6-3   Representative examples of peptide
hormones and hormones derived from amino acids.
Thyroxine is synthesized from tyrosine.

effects. Note, and compare with Figure 6-2, that, while all primary and most
secondary tissues release other hormones, the tertiary tissues cause the
ultimate physiological response. As shown in the figure, the adrenal medulla and the pancreas are notable exceptions. The adrenal medulla responds to sympathetic input to secrete epinephrine as a response to stress.
The pancreas secretes insulin and other hormones in response to circulating levels of glucose (Chapter 3), even though it is also influenced by growth
hormone. The chemical structures of four hormones given in Table 6-1 are
shown in Figure 6-3.

Table 6-2 details five important steroid hormones. All steroid hormones
are DNA enhancers and, in addition to their specific effects, have some
degree of either glucose synthesizing effects (glucocortical) or sodium re-
taining effects (mineralocortical). As a result of being glucocorticoids and
mineralocorticoids, steroids may produce undesirable physiological effects
such as: potassium depletion, weight gain, excessive mental stimulation,
osteoporosis (bone resorption), adrenal atrophy, and even the induction of
diabetes. This may occur as a result of the presence of a higher than normal
amount of the hormone or exposure to the hormone for a prolonged period
of time. Such conditions may occur in steroid diseases (e.g., Cushing's syndrome), steroid intake abuse (e.g., in the case of athletes who take steroids to
greatly increase their capabilities), and steroid therapy (e.g., among patients
treated for chronic arthritis). Certain steroids such as cortisol, and its synthetic cousins, are known for their ability to suppress the inflammatory

**TABLE 6-2    Steroid Hormones***

| Hormone | Molecular Weight | Source | Target | Mechanism | Effect |
|---|---|---|---|---|---|
| Cortisol | 360 | Adrenal cortex | Many tissues | DNA enhancer | Glucose synthesis: anti-inflammatory |
| Aldosterone | 371 | Adrenal cortex | Kidneys | DNA enhancer | Sodium retention and potassium excretion |
| Estradiol | 272 | Ovary | Female organs | DNA enhancer | Sexual maturation of female |
| Testosterone | 288 | Testis | Male organs | DNA enhancer | Sexual maturation of male |
| Progesterone | 315 | Ovary | Uterus | DNA enhancer | Preparation, continuance of pregnancy |

*This list is selective. The reader should consult other texts for other hormones in this classification.

response (discussed in Chapter 8). Figure 6-4 shows the structures of four steroids that are metabolically derived from cholesterol. Although the molecular differences among the steroids are quite small, the effects produced can be quite different in specificity and degree.

The two cyclic nucleotide hormones (Table 6-3, Figure 6-4) are the intracellular second messengers. Other second messengers are calcium ions and phosphoinositides. The latter seems to be a messenger system within the plasma membrane of a cell. The cyclic nucleotides generally produce opposing effects within a cell and operate by amplifying their signal by a cascade mechanism, which is discussed later in this chapter.

Table 6-4 lists four eicosanoid hormones and their effects. Two of their structures are shown in Figure 6-4. Eicosanoids are made from long-chain fatty acids and produce a variety of physiological responses that also often oppose one another. Eicosanoids are local hormones.

## Plasma Membrane Binding Hormones and Their Receptors: Mechanisms

Hormones that bind to plasma membrane receptors (see Figure 6-1) can initiate a variety of intracellular events. In speaking of a *targeted* cell for such hormones, it is meant that a particular cell possesses a protein capable of binding to a specific hormone. Not all cells have receptors for every hormone. Those that do can produce different responses to the same hormone. That is what causes the specificity and diversity of hormones. An example of a receptor protein for insulin was shown in Figure 3-27. It causes intracellular effects by altering the activity of the enzyme tyrosine kinase. The tyrosine kinase is part of the structure of the receptor protein itself. It brings about effects such as increased uptake of glucose, mobilization of lipids into the bloodstream and the active transport of amino acids into cells.

Most receptor proteins, however, cause activation or deactivation of enzymes that make the secondary messengers cyclic adenosine monophosphate (cAMP) and cyclic guanosine monophosphate (cGMP). A G (guanosine) protein acts as an intermediary in the process (Figure 6-5). When the hormone binds to its receptor protein it brings about uptake of the nucleotide guanosine triphosphate (GTP) in the α-subunit of a G protein. As this occurs, the α-subunit is detached from the other subunits and diffuses to the membrane enzyme adenylate cyclase. The α-subunit binds to

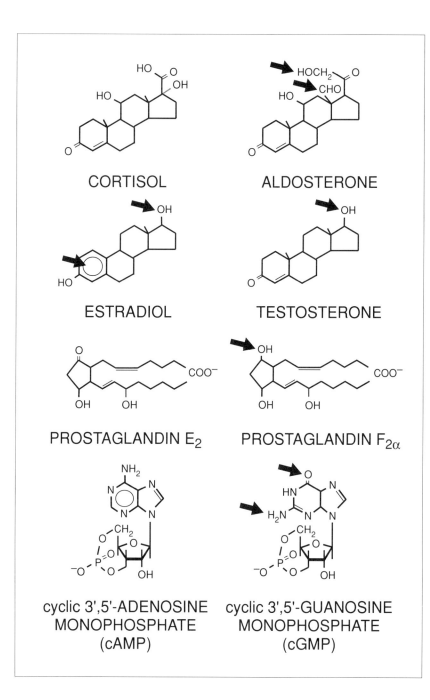

**FIGURE 6-4** Representative steroid hormones (top four), eicosanoid hormones (prostaglandins), and second messenger hormones (cyclic nucleotides).
Arrows indicate functional group differences within each class.

the enzyme and either stimulates it (if it comes from a $G_S$ protein) or inhibits it (if it comes from a $G_I$ protein). Most hormones, however, operate through $G_S$ proteins, to stimulate adenylate cyclase. In the next chapter, it will be shown that many neurotransmitters operate through $G_I$ proteins.

Adenylate cyclase causes the formation of the second messenger cAMP. The corresponding cGMP enzyme is guanylate cyclase. Cyclic AMP and cGMP produce cellular effects by means of a cascade mechanism, which essentially involves an amplification of the signal or message carried by the extracellular hormone. This means that the molecule representing the "message" causes the production of many more molecules that affect a response to the message. This is accomplished with several enzymes in the cascade. Figure 6-6 shows the cascade produced by epinephrine to increase

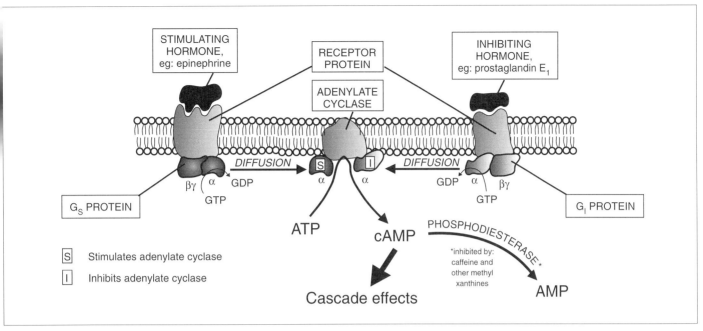

**FIGURE 6-5**  Mechanisms of plasma membrane hormone receptor protein reacitons.

The stimulatory mechanism (shown at left) is one in which the receptor protein binds to a stimulatory G protein (or $G_S$). This protein (consisting of α-, β-, and γ subunits) normally is bound to guanosine diphosphate (GDP, a nucleotide), at its α-subunit. When the hormone receptor protein binds to it, it releases GDP and takes up guanosine triphosphate (GTP). As this occurs, the GTP–α-subunit complex is released from the other two G protein subunits and diffuses to the nearest adenylate cyclase enzyme (bound to the plasma membrane), binds to it, and causes its activation. The activated adenylate cyclase catalyzes the formation of cAMP (from ATP), which begins the cascade mechanism of hormone effects. The inhibitory mechanism (shown at the right) occurs less frequently with hormones. It is similar to the stimulatory mechanism, except that an inhibitory G protein (or $G_I$) is involved. The α-subunit of the G protein shuts down (or inhibits) the adenylate cyclase. A cytoplasmic phosphodiesterase eventually hydrolyzes cAMP to AMP. Cyclic GMP is activated and broken down in a somewhat similar manner. (Adapted from Mathews CK, and van Holde KE. *Biochemistry.* Redwood City, CA: Benjamin/Cummings, 1990;799.)

**TABLE 6-3   Cyclic Nucleotide Hormones (Second Messengers)**

| Hormone | Molecular Weight | Source | Target | Mechanism | Effect |
|---|---|---|---|---|---|
| cAMP | 329 | PM receptor | Various intracellular | Cascade | Often stimultory |
| cGMP | 345 | PM receptor | Various intracellular | Cascade | Often inhibitory, visual transduction |

Key: cAMP, cyclic adenosine 3′,5′-monophosphate; cGMP, cyclic guanosine 3′,5′-monophosphate.

**TABLE 6-4   Eicosanoid Hormones***

| Hormone | Molecular weight | Source | Target | Mechanism | Effect |
|---|---|---|---|---|---|
| Prostaglandin $E_2$ | 352 | Ubiquitous cells | Local cells | Membrane receptor, second messenger | Relaxes smooth muscles; causes inflammation |
| Prostaglandin $F_{2\alpha}$ | 355 | Ubiquitous cells | Local cells | Membrane receptor, second messenger | Contracts smooth muscles |
| Leucotriene $E_4$ | 454 | White blood cells, lungs | Local cells | Membrane receptor, second messenger | Exudation of plasma |
| Thromboxane $B_2$ | 370 | Platelets, others | Local cells | Membrane receptor, second messenger | Contracts smooth muscle |

*This list is selective; the reader should consult other texts for other hormones in this class.

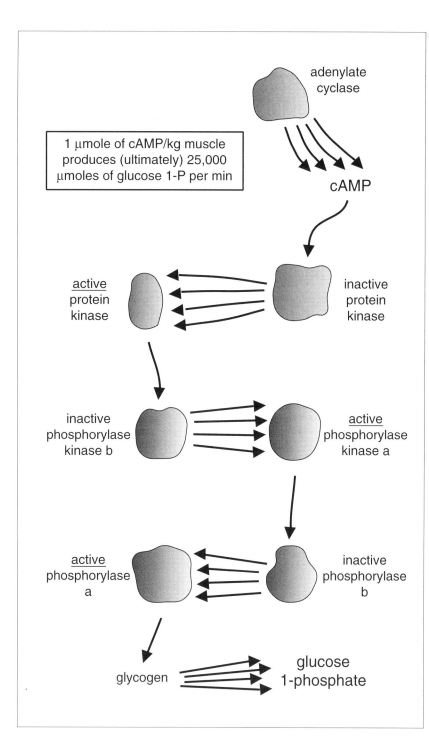

1 μmole of cAMP/kg muscle produces (ultimately) 25,000 μmoles of glucose 1-P per min

adenylate cyclase

cAMP

active protein kinase

inactive protein kinase

inactive phosphorylase kinase b

active phosphorylase kinase a

active phosphorylase a

inactive phosphorylase b

glycogen

glucose 1-phosphate

**FIGURE 6-6   The cascade mechanism.**
Many cascade mechanisms begin with cAMP or cGMP and involve the activation of several intermediate enzymes by adding phosphate (phosphorylation) to inactive enzymes by using a kinase enzyme. Cyclic nucleotides activate the first kinase. The particular example shown is for the formation of glucose-1-phosphate from the binding of the hormone adrenaline (epinephrine) to its receptor protein. (Adapted from McGilvery RW, and Goldstein GW. *Biochemistry, a Functional Approach,* 3rd ed. Philadelphia: WB Saunders, 1983;515.)

the amount of intracellular glucose participating in the Embden-Meyerhof (E-M) pathway (Chapter 3). In other words, it increases the amount of energy produced by a cell. In the mechanism, cAMP activates a protein kinase (an enzyme causing the addition of phosphate groups). The active protein kinase, in turn, activates a phosphorylase kinase, which in turn activates a third enzyme, phosphorylase. Phosphorylase (see Chapter 3) causes the formation of glucose 1-phosphate from glycogen stores. Glucose 1-phosphate is a precursor to glucose 6-phosphate, which participates in glycolysis (i.e., the E-M pathway, see Chapter 3).

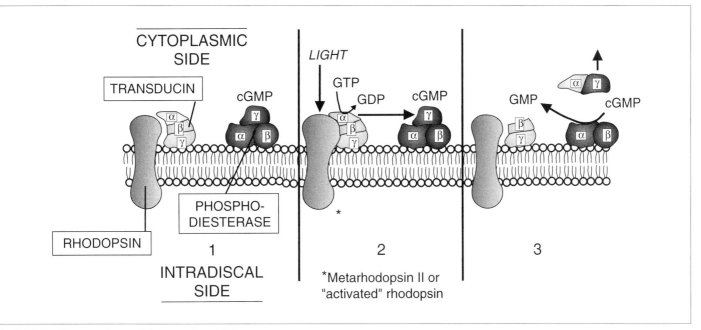

**FIGURE 6-7    Disc membrane, light receptor protein transduction mechanism.**

Similar to the hormone receptor protein mechanism, light activates rhodopsin and, ultimately, affects the level of a cyclic nucleotide. On the cytoplasmic side of each disc: rhodopsin (the receptor protein), transducin (the G protein), and guanylate phosphodiesterase (instead of a cyclase) are located in close proximity (shown at 1) on the disc membrane. When light strikes a rhodopsin molecule, the molecular rearrangement of vitamin A (to an unprotonated Schiff base) and the protein conformation of the opsin portion (to metarhodopsin II) cause close contact with transducin. As before (see Figure 6-5), the α-subunit of transducin takes up GTP, breaks away from the other subunits, and diffuses to the phosphodiesterase molecule (shown at 2). The α-subunit of transducin binds to the γ-subunit of the phosphodiesterase, causing it to be released from the enzyme. The release activates the enzyme bringing about the catalysis of a cGMP to GMP. (Adapted from Stryer L. *Biochemistry*, 3rd ed. New York: WH Freeman and Co., 1988;1034.)

The number of molecules produced is amplified many times with the activation of each enzyme. McGilvery and Goldstein (1983) estimate that 1 μmol of cAMP (itself amplified from adenylate cyclase by the hormone epinephrine) will cause the synthesis of 25,000 μmol of glucose 1-phosphate per minute. Similar mechanisms of production and cascade, involving guanylate cyclase, exist for cGMP. Both cAMP and cGMP are inactivated to AMP and GMP, respectively, by separate phosphodiesterase enzymes (see Figure 6-5). Phosphodiesterases are inhibited by methyl xanthines, notably caffeine and theophylline, substances found in significant concentrations in coffee, certain soft drinks, chocolate, and tea. Accordingly, the increase in the amounts of second messengers, particularly cAMP, accounts for central nervous system stimulation, cardiac stimulation, and gastric motility when these substances are consumed (Rall, 1985). Although these enzymes are present in the eye, vision is not improved by drinking coffee or eating chocolate.

## Light Transduction: A cGMP Mechanism

In Chapter 1 the molecular properties of rhodopsin are described. The role of rhodopsin in vision is similar to that of a receptor protein for a hormone. However, light replaces the hormone and the G protein associated with rhodopsin causes activation of a phosphodiesterase, rather than a cyclase. The G protein, known as *transducin*, functions like other G proteins, since it incorporates GTP (while removing guanosine diphosphate [GDP]) when it interacts with the activated rhodopsin molecule. The α-subunit of transducin detaches and diffuses to an inactive phosphodiesterase for cGMP. The α-subunit of transducin binds to the γ-subunit of phosphodiesterase, causing that subunit to leave the enzyme. This action activates the enzyme, which quickly lowers the concentration of cGMP in the cytoplasm of photoreceptor outer segments (Figure 6-7). Note that the respective orientations of rhodopsin (receptor protein), transducin (G protein), and phosphodiesterase (enzyme) molecules seem inverted when compared to

Figure 6-5. It should be kept in mind, however, that rod discs are internal and that the orientation must be inverted if the mechanism is to affect the photoreceptor cytoplasm.

These questions arise: Why is cGMP important for vision? Why does ultimately lowering the concentration of cGMP translate into a perception of light in the brain? The answers lie in the controlled operation of the flow of sodium ions into the photoreceptor at the outer segment (both rods and cones) and out again at the inner segment. This is *the dark current,* so named due to its flow being maximal in the dark. The inward flow of sodium ions is controlled by gate proteins at the outer segment and the outward flow, by Na,K-ATPase at the inner segment (Figure 6-8).

While the activity of Na,K-ATPase is virtually constant, the open channels through the gate proteins require that cGMP be bound to the gate proteins in order to remain open. When the concentration of cGMP is lowered through the activity of cGMP phosphodiesterase, cGMP leaves the gate proteins, which close and begin to interrupt the flow of sodium. The activity of phosphodiesterase is controlled by the effects of light on the rhodopsin-transducin-phosphodiesterase cascade. When the sodium influx is interrupted, sodium efflux continues and the departing positively charged sodium ions cause the photoreceptors to acquire a greater negative charge. In effect, the cells hyperpolarize. This hyperpolarization is unusual

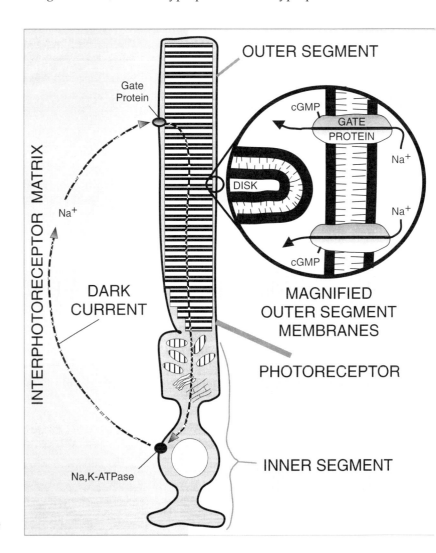

**FIGURE 6-8  The dark current in photoreceptors.**
The current is made up of the flow of sodium ions cycled between photoreceptors and the interphotoreceptor matrix. Sodium ions enter each photoreceptor's outer segment through gate proteins to which cGMP is bound. The ions travel through the cell and exit at the inner segment by the "pumping" activity of Na,K-ATPase. When cGMP is not bound to the gate protein, the sodium ion pore in the center of each gate protein is closed.

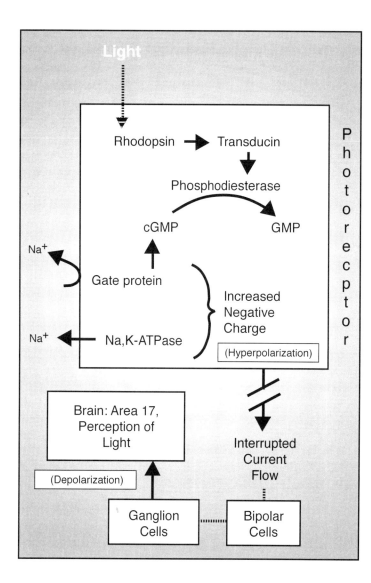

**FIGURE 6-9  Complete diagram of visual transduction.**
The large white box represents events that occur in Figure
6-7 and cause the interruption of dark current (Figure 6-8).
The interrupted dark current hyperpolarizes photoreceptors and actually causes bipolar cells to depolarize,
which in turn, brings about the depolarization of ganglion
cells. The signal conveyed by the ganglion cells is carried to
area 17 of the brain, where it is perceived as light. The
highly unusual hyperpolarization in photoreceptors
(and, sometimes, bipolar cells also) is discussed in
Chapter 7.

since it stops the flow of current to the ganglion cells of the retina, causing
the ganglion cells to discharge. The discharge to area 17 of the brain is
perceived as light. The entire visual transduction process is diagrammed in
Figure 6-9.

## Graves' Disease

Hyperthyroidism (Graves' disease) is a condition in which the thyroid
gland releases excessive amounts of its hormones, triiodothyronine ($T_3$)
and thyroxine (tetraiodothyronine, $T_4$). First described in 1786 by Parry, it
was later associated with a description by Graves in 1835. The nonocular
symptoms of the disease include nervousness, irritability, fatigue, weight
loss, heat sensitivity, heart palpitations, and weakness. All of these symptoms result from the increased metabolic rate induced by greater than normal amounts of circulating $T_3$ and $T_4$ in the bloodstream. The thyroid gland
is usually enlarged.

Approximately 30% to 65% of hyperthyroid patients have ocular symptoms (Char, 1990a). The eyes are often proptosed or partially pushed forward from their sockets, a condition known as exophthalmos. This includes
retraction of the upper eyelids and difficulty in being able to close the eyes.

The eyes are pushed forward by a tissue build-up around the extraocular muscles. In extreme cases this build-up can result in corneal drying (from the inability to close the eyes) and optic nerve damage (possibly due to compression of the nerve by the extraocular tissue build-up).

Graves' disease results from the existence of one or more proteins that act as if they were the thyroid-stimulating hormone (TSH, or thyrotropin) released by the anterior pituitary (see Figure 6-2). The proteins are, in fact, antibodies (see Chapter 8)—called: *thyroid-stimulating immunoglobulins (TSI)* (Utiger, 1987). These antibodies regard the thyroid gland as a foreign tissue (antigen) and bind to it as a means of tagging the thyroid for immunological rejection. However, in the process they happen to bind to the receptor protein for TSH, and, since there are more of them, they cause an increase in the circulation of $T_3$ and $T_4$ (Figure 6-10). The only direct ocular effect produced by the increase of $T_3$ and $T_4$ is lid retraction (Utiger, 1987). This is due to the effect of $T_3$ and $T_4$ on the sympathetic innervation of the lids (Char, 1990b). The swelling of the extraocular muscle tissues (causing proptosis) is considered to be an infiltrative event. It is related to an immunochemical mechanism and will be considered in Chapter 8.

## DNA Binding Hormones: Mechanism

Second messengers are able to affect RNA transcription, and ultimately, protein synthesis. However, the influence of steroid hormones and thyroid hormones on RNA transcription is better understood. Steroid hormones and endocrine hormones from the thyroid gland ($T_3$ and $T_4$) ultimately bind to DNA enhancers (Alberts et al., 1989) (see Figure 6-1). However, this is accomplished only after the hormone has entered the cell and is initially bound to a protein receptor located in the cytoplasm. In fact, it is the receptor protein itself that actually binds to the DNA enhancer. The general structure of DNA-binding steroid receptors is indicated in Figure 6-11. The action and conformational change induced in the receptor protein by the

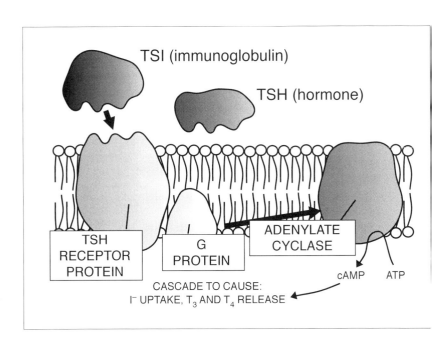

**FIGURE 6-10　Plasma membrane, hormone receptor protein reaction mechanism in the thyroid gland.** Here, in Graves' disease, a thyroid-stimulating immunoglobulin (TSI) mimics the response achieved by the thyroid-stimulating hormone (TSH). The result is an increase in the release and circulation of $T_3$ and $T_4$.

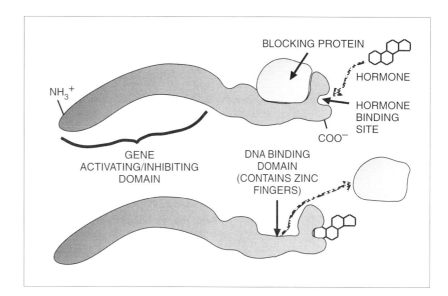

**FIGURE 6-11** Steroid and thyroid hormone receptor proteins.

A blocking protein is normally bound to the DNA-binding domain of the protein. When the hormone binds to the protein, it causes the release of the blocking protein. (Adapted from Alberts B, Bray D, Lewis J, Raff M, Roberts K, and Watson JD. *Molecular Biology of the Cell,* 2nd ed. New York: Garland, 1989;691.)

hormone's binding causes the release of a blocking protein from the DNA-binding domain. This action enables the receptor protein–hormone complex to bind to the appropriate enhancer site on DNA after diffusion into the cell nucleus.

After this takes place, the enhancer region may influence either the initiation or the inhibition of gene transcription—and ultimately protein synthesis—by close contact with the promoter region or with RNA polymerase in that region (Figure 6-12). In the figure, a steroid hormone–receptor protein complex binds to an enhancer while RNA polymerase binds to a nearby promoter. In this case, close contact or binding of the gene-activating region of the receptor protein signals the RNA polymerase to begin transcription. Such enhanced or increased transcription causes the cell to make larger quantities of specific kinds of proteins, usually enzymes.

An example of this mechanism is what takes place with the steroid hormone aldosterone (see Table 6-2, Figure 6-4). Aldosterone causes retention of sodium ions and loss of potassium ions in the kidneys as a means of maintaining specific ion concentrations in the blood (mineralocorticoid

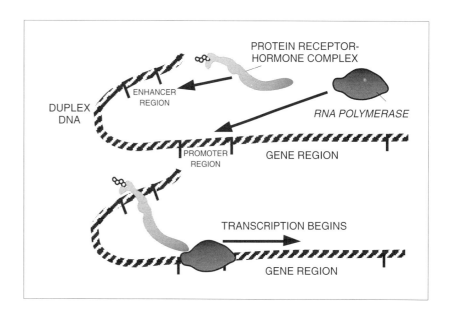

**FIGURE 6-12** Hormone-enhancer mechanism for RNA transcription.

When the intracellular hormone-binding protein complex is formed, it diffuses to the nucleus where it binds to a specific enhancer region on DNA. The gene-activating or -inhibiting domain extends to the promoter region (lower part of figure) where it causes transcription to begin or prevents it from occurring.

activity). Without such control an individual would die in a matter of days. Verrey et al. (1989) found that aldosterone induces a rapid increase in the rate of Na,K-ATPase gene transcription in cultured kidney cells. Na,K-ATPase is responsible for transport of sodium and potassium ions, and, therefore, an increase in this enzyme's synthesis supports such a kidney mechanism (Figure 6-13). This is so since raising the concentration of this enzyme (via enhanced synthesis using aldosterone) maintains the required transport of ions in the kidney.

In the eye, steroid and thyroid hormones alter protein synthesis, both positively and negatively, to affect cellular function by such mechanisms (DNA binding). A practical example is the increased lid retraction mentioned in the hyperthyroidism of Graves' disease as a result of high levels of $T_3$ and $T_4$. Normally, however, $T_3$ and $T_4$ stimulate optimal metabolism (i.e., via enzyme synthesis) in all ocular cells. Although, clinically, both natural and synthesized steroid hormones are better known for their ability to inhibit inflammatory reactions in the eye (Chapter 8), they can also produce some undesirable effects in ocular tissues.

In the cornea, there can be an increase in corneal thickness with the use of topically applied steroids as well as some natural steroids when present at elevated levels (Soni, 1980). The latter occurs, for example, with pregnant women who have high levels of estriol and pregnanediol (two steroids related to estradiol and aldosterone in structure). More serious, however, are the posterior subcapsular cataracts in the lens associated with the prolonged use of steroids to treat nonocular diseases such as rheumatoid arthritis. Mayman et al. (1979) reported that the enzyme Na,K-ATPase is "inhibited" in lens tissues with the therapeutic use of dexamethasone (an aldosterone-like synthetic steroid). Presumably (since it has not been adequately demonstrated), these steroids are acting to inhibit the synthesis of Na,K-ATPase by preventing the transcription of mRNA for Na,K-ATPase. This action is exactly the opposite of the positive enhancement by aldosterone.

In effect, some steroids can cause swelling of newly formed lens fiber cells just below the posterior capsule. This swelling represents the initiation of a cataract. It occurs from the decreased ability of the cells to transport sodium and postassium ions. This action is likewise related to the steroidal decrease

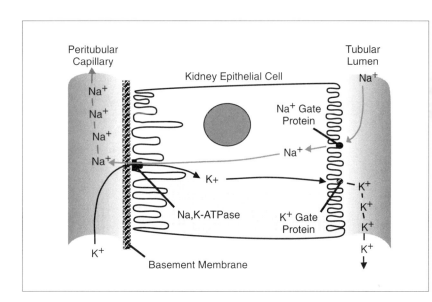

**FIGURE 6-13** Cross section of kidney epithelial cell with peritubular capillary (*left*) and collecting duct or tubular lumen (*right*).

The formation of urine in the tubular lumen is partially realized by extracting sodium and releasing potassium into the tubular lumen. In the process, the bloodstream regains sodium and loses potassium by having these ions pass through the epithelial cell. The action is catalyzed by Na,K-ATPase as well as the facilitation provided by sodium and potassium gate proteins. This action has some similarities to the formation of aqueous from blood in the ciliary body (see Figure 2-19).

in mRNA specific for the synthesis of Na,K-ATPase. It results finally in the osmotic inclusion of water. Other explanations, such as binding of steroids to lens proteins, have been offered (Urban and Cottier, 1986), but no proof of any alternate mechanism has been given. If synthetic steroids cause cataracts, why are cataracts not caused by high levels of natural steroid hormones such as the example of pregnancy just given? Three reasons may be presented: (1) the specific effects of a particular steroid on an enhancer, (2) the level or concentration of the steroid in a tissue, and (3) the duration of steroid stimulation during which a given steroid is present in a tissue. Table 6-5 shows a comparison of three steroids: their body fluid concentrations, time in those fluids, and ocular effects. As can be seen, the duration of exposure can be more meaningful than the concentration, whereas the particular steroid determines its ultimate ocular effects on ocular tissues. Although the natural steroid pregnanediol can cause corneal swelling (and difficulties with wearing contact lenses), the condition is temporary. Prolonged use of the synthetic steroid prednisone, however, can produce permanent cataracts. The use of synthetic steroids can also raise intraocular pressure. Although the mechanism for this is presently not understood, evidence suggests that it is an enhancer mechanism (Jaanus, 1989).

## Paracrine Hormones

Paracrine hormones are released by cells in the immediate vicinity of their site of action. This is why they are called *local hormones.* Their effectiveness is also limited by the fact that they are very rapidly destroyed after being released. Eicosanoids (see Table 6-4) are the principal members of this class, but some small peptides and amino acid derivatives seem to fall within this classification also. An example of the latter is histamine, derived from the amino acid histidine. Histamine signals the release of white blood cells from blood vessels to an infected tissue. Here, however, we concentrate on eicosanoids.

Eicosanoids are formed initially at the cell's plasma membrane as shown in Figure 6-14. Those cells that make prostaglandins do so by cannibalizing arachidonic and other highly unsaturated long-chain fatty acids from their

TABLE 6-5    Steroids, Their Body Fluid Concentrations, Duration of Presence, and Ocular Effects

| Steroid | Present During | Fluid Level ($\mu$g/dL) | Duration | Ocular Effect |
|---|---|---|---|---|
| Cortisol | Lifetime | 23[*] | Lifelong | None |
| Pregnanediol | Pregnancy | 206[*] | 24 wk[†] | Corneal swelling |
| Prednisone | Arthritis treatment | 35[‡] | 192 wk | Cataracts |
| Prednisone | Ocular inflammation treatment | 100[§] | <6 wk | None |

[*]Levels approach this amount in blood plasma (see Tietz, 1986).

[†]Last 24 weeks of pregnancy.

[‡]Levels in blood plasma for treatment of rheumatoid arthritis (see Stubbs, 1975).

[§]Levels in the aqueous humor of rabbits (see Schoenwald and Boltralik, 1979).

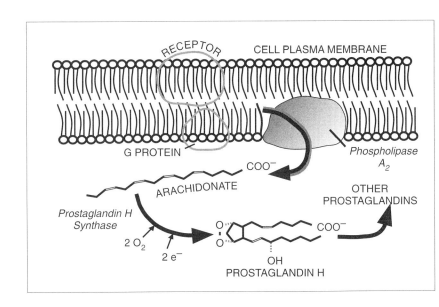

**FIGURE 6-14    The formation of prostaglandins from plasma membrane lipids.**
Arachidonate and other highly unsaturated fatty acids are removed from membrane phospholipids by hydrolysis with phospholipase A₂. A receptor protein–G protein complex (outlines) may stimulate the phospholipase A₂. These fatty acids are cyclized, oxygenated, and reduced by prostaglandin synthase (an enzyme complex with three separate catalytic activities) to prostaglandin H. Note the requirement for oxygen and a source of electrons. The H form of the prostaglandin then becomes the substrate for catalysis to other prostaglandins.

plasma membranes. This is accomplished by breaking fatty acid ester bonds on phospholipids in the membranes with the enzyme phospholipase A₂. However, this process may also be assisted by a linked receptor protein—G protein complex, which activates the phospholipase A₂ more strongly. This means that an outside signaling molecule (not necessarily a hormone) can increase the production of eicosanoids. In the cytoplasm, the released fatty acid is cyclized, oxygenated, and then reduced by a multifunctional enzyme, *prostaglandin synthase* (also called a *cyclooxygenase*). This enzyme requires both molecular oxygen and a source of electrons to transform the fatty acid to the initial prostaglandin H.

*Prostaglandin synthase is inhibited by aspirin.* Since some prostaglandins cause inflammatory responses, this explains how aspirin produces an anti-inflammatory effect as a medication (see Chapter 8). Other prostaglandins (and related compounds known as *thromboxanes*) are formed enzymatically from prostaglandin H. Still another enzyme, *lipoxygenase*, forms an additional class of eicosanoids, called *leukotrienes*, from arachidonate and similarly released fatty acids. The leukotrienes are oxygenated, but not cyclized as the prostaglandins are.

When prostaglandins and related eicosanoids are released to affect nearby cells, they bind to receptor proteins on those cells to increase or decrease the levels of second messengers located there. This is accomplished in the same manner as that of an endocrine hormone (see Figure 6-5). Likewise, the effects produced may be either stimulatory or inhibitory. There are at least 13 different prostaglandins and thromboxanes as well as 11 different leukotrienes that can be formed from three major long-chain, unsaturated fatty acids (Mayes, 1985). The physiological effects produced by these hormones, like those of endocrine hormones, are quite varied. They include control of the ion composition of the blood and of blood pressure, modulation of lung functions, influence on cell proliferation, control of the inflammatory reaction, mediation of gastrointestinal functions, wound healing, and even endocrine function itself (Watkins et al., 1989).

Eicosanoids are known to affect the function of virtually every tissue in the eye (Bito and Stjernschantz, 1989). The detailed mechanisms of these functions have not been adequately described as yet. Mittag (1989) provides some evidence that the iris and ciliary muscles are relaxed by prostaglandin $E_{2\alpha}$ ($PGE_{2\alpha}$). Candia et al. (1989) indicated that $PGF_{2\alpha}$ stimulates production of intraocular fluid by the ciliary epithelium. Neither investigator indicates which local cells may be providing the prostaglandins or the reason for their release. However, Miranda and Bito (1989) have shown, from a series of investigations by others, that trauma (injury) to both the cornea and the iris itself releases prostaglandins to affect the miosis (closing) of the iris sphincter muscle. This is a natural protective reaction to injury.

In the retina, Vinores et al. (1992) have demonstrated that PGE can cause breakdown of the blood-retina barrier by opening the tight junctions between vascular endothelial cells. Such a process brings about macular edema. This fills the retinal macula with fluid and can cause visual blurring. Trauma to the retina can be a cause of the release of prostaglandins here. In fact, response to trauma is a common cause of prostaglandin release in ocular and nonocular tissues. The mediation of prostaglandins in ocular inflammation is discussed in Chapter 8.

It is important that the influence of prostaglandins on the ciliary body and the production of aqueous fluid is understood, since this has direct application to the treatment of glaucoma. Although Candia et al. (1989) have found a stimulation of aqueous production by $PGF_{2\alpha}$, Alm and Villumsen (1989) reported no effect but a probable increase in the uveoscleral outflow to lower intraocular pressure (IOP). The uveoscleral pathway is a second pathway for the exit of aqueous fluid. Selen et al. (1991) have indicated that both an increase in uveoscleral outflow and aqueous production occur. However, the increase in uveoscleral outflow is greater, resulting in a net decrease in IOP. The specific biochemical mechanism, other than involving membrane receptors and a cascade, is not known.

## Summary

Hormones are chemical messengers that integrate the cooperative intercellular functions of humans and animals. They are concerned with such functions as growth, metabolism, sexual function, and inflammatory reactions. In the eye, hormones assist in the smooth functioning of the visual process. A hormonelike mechanism is involved in visual transduction. There are five chemical classes of hormones: peptides, derived amino acids, cyclic nucleotides, steroids, and eicosanoids. There are four functional classes of hormones: endocrine hormones that bind to a cellular surface, endocrine hormones that bind to DNA, intracellular hormones (second messengers), and paracrine hormones that bind to a cellular surface.

All hormones have receptor proteins, either at the cell surface or within the cell cytoplasm. Receptor proteins *at the cell surface* react with G proteins and either activate (usually) or inhibit an enzyme that forms or breaks down cyclic nucleotides. This process activates or inhibits a cascade mechanism via the cyclic nucleotide. Receptor proteins *in the cytoplasm* bind to the hormone and carry it to the cell nucleus, where the complex binds to a DNA enhancer. There are receptors for many types of hormones in the eye. They cause a variety of responses, including lid retraction, cessation of inflammation, uptake of glucose into cells (nourishment), and changes in intraocular pressure. It is also possible that these hormones can induce corneal swelling, cataract formation, and inflammation. How hormones affect the eye depends on the type and concentration of hormones and on how long ocular tissues are exposed to those hormones.

## References

Alberts B, Bray D, Lewis J, Raff M, Roberts K, and Watson JD. *Molecular Biology of the Cell*, 2nd ed. New York: Garland, 1989;690–693.

Alm A, and Villumsen J. Effects of topically applied $PGE_{2\alpha}$ and its isopropylester on normal and glaucomatous human eyes. *In* Bito LZ, and Stjernschantz J (eds.). *The Ocular Effects of Prostaglandins and Other Eicosanoids.* New York: Alan R. Liss, 1989;447–458.

Bito LZ, and Stjernschantz J (eds). *The Ocular Effects of Prostaglandins and Other Eicosanoids.* New York: Alan R. Liss, 1989.

Candia OA, Chu T-C, and Alvarez L. Prostaglandins and transepithelial ionic transport. *In* Bito LZ, and Stjernschantz J (eds). *The Ocular Effects of Prostaglandins and Other Eicosanoids.* New York: Alan R. Liss, 1989;149–154.

Char DH. *Thyroid Eye Disease*, 2nd ed. New York: Churchill Livingstone, 1990a;5–19.

Char DH. *Thyroid Eye Disease,* 2nd ed. New York: Churchill Livingstone, 1990b; 99.

Graves RJ. Newly observed affection of the thyroid gland in females. *London Med Surg J* 1835;7:516–520.

Jaanus SD. Anti-inflammatory drugs. *In* Bartlett JD, and Jaanus SD (eds). *Clinical Ocular Pharmacology*, 2nd ed. Boston: Butterworths, 1989;163–197.

Mathews CK, and van Holde KE. *Biochemistry.* Redwood City, CA: Benjamin/Cummings, 1990;637–641.

Mayes PA. Metabolism of lipids: I. Fatty acids. *In* Martin DW, Mayes PA, Rodwell VW, and Granner DK (eds). *Harper's Review of Biochemistry*, 20th ed. Los Altos, CA: Lange, 1985;221–241.

Mayman CI, Miller D, and Tijerina ML. In vitro production of steroid cataract in bovine lens: Part II, Measurement of sodium-potassium adenosine triphosphatase activity. *Acta Ophthalmol* 1979;57:1107–1117.

McGilvery RW, and Goldstein GW. *Biochemistry: A Functional Approach.* Philadelphia: WB Saunders, 1983;515.

Miranda OC, and Bito LZ. The putative and demonstrated miotic effects of prostaglandins in mammals. *In* Bito LZ and Stjernschantz (eds). *The Ocular Effects of Prostaglandins and Other Eicosanoids.* New York: Alan R. Liss, 1989;171–195.

Mittag TW. Signal transduction systems for prostaglandins in the iris and ciliary body. *In* Bito LZ, and Stjernschantz J (eds).*The Ocular Effects of Prostaglandins and Other Eicosanoids.* New York: Alan R. Liss, 1989;139–148.

Parry CH. Enlargement of thyroid gland in connection with enlargement or palpitation of the heart. In *Collections from Unpublished Writings of Late Caleb Hillier Parry,* vol 2. London: Underwoods, 1825;2.

Rall TW. The methylxanthines. *In* Gilman AG, Goodman LS, Rall TW, and Murad F (eds). *The Pharmacological Basis of Therapeutics.* New York: MacMillan, 1985;589–603.

Schoenwald RD, and Boltralik JJ. A bioavailability comparison in rabbits of two steroids formulated as high-viscosity gels and reference aqueous preparations. *Invest Ophthalmol Vis Sci* 1979;18:61–66.

Selen G, Karlsson M, Astin M, Stjernschantz J, and Resul B. Effects of PhXA34 and PhDG100A, two phenyl substituted prostaglandin esters, on aqueous humor dynamics and microcirculation in the monkey eye. *Invest Ophthalmol Vis Sci* 1991;32:988.

Soni PS. Effects of oral contraceptive steroids on the thickness of human cornea. *Am J Optom Physiol Optics* 1980;57:825–334.

Stubbs SS. Corticosteroids and bioavailability. *Transplant Proc* 1975;7:11–19.

Tietz NW (ed). *Textbook of Clinical Chemistry,* 1st ed. Philadelphia: WB Saunders, 1986;1820, 1842.

Urban RC, and Cottier E. Corticosteroid-induced cataracts. *Surv Ophthalmol* 1986;31:102–110.

Utiger RD. Hyperthyroidism. *In* Green WL (ed.) *The Thyroid.* New York: Elsevier, 1987;161–162.

Verrey F, Kraehenbuhl JP, and Rossier BC. Aldosterone induces a rapid increase in the rate of Na,K-ATPase gene transcription in cultured kidney cells. *Molec Endocrinol* 1989;3:1369–1376.

Vinores SA, Harsha, S, and Campachiaro PA. An adenosine agonist and prostaglandin $E_1$ cause breakdown of the blood-retinal barrier by opening tight junctions between vascular endothelial cells. *Invest Ophthalmol Vis Sci* 1992;33:1870–1878.

Watkins WO, Peterson MB, and Fletcher JR (eds). *Prostaglandins in Clinical Practice.* New York: Raven, 1989.

# Chapter 7

# Neurotransmitters and Neurotransmission

## Review of Neurotransmission

Neurotransmission is a highly efficient and rapid mechanism for sending messages to and from the brain and other body tissues. In the eye, it facilitates such functions as tear secretion, miosis, maintenance of intraocular pressure, and the very act of seeing. Just outside the eye it mediates eye movement, blinking, and lid closure. The transmission of nervous signals throughout the body is accomplished by a combination of two biochemical processes: the transport of cations through membranes (creating the action potential in nerves) and the diffusion of neurotransmitter molecules from one neuron to the next or to a muscle cell (as occurs at the synaptic cleft). Neurotransmitters function just like discrete hormones. That is, they have hormone action but only within the area of a synaptic cleft. Like hormones, each neurotransmitter binds to a receptor protein that produces either: (1) a continuation of an action potential (stimulation), (2) prevention of an action potential (inhibition), or (3) muscle contraction (stimulation). The details are explained further on. It is also important to understand the nature of the action potential that leads up to neurotransmitter release.

An action potential, unlike electricity flowing through a wire by means of electron movement, results from the rapid, sequential flow of sodium ions into a cell and potassium ions outward. A cell normally has a relatively high *internal* concentration of potassium (140 mM vs 5 mM externally) and a relatively high *external* concentration of sodium (145 mM vs ~10 mM internally). The combination of these concentration differences creates a potential difference across cell membranes of approximately 60 mV (in some neurons the potential may be as high as 90 mV) with the inside of the cell being negative. The action potential begins when separate gate proteins for sodium and potassium open in sequence to allow the cations to flow through the membrane. (Figure 7-1). The potential difference, shown in the figure as $-64$ mV (at time zero), is established and maintained by the constant pumping activity of Na,K-ATPase (Chapter 2), as well as a very small leakage of both ions across the membrane. At time zero, a wave of depolarization reaches the membrane from either an adjacent section of nerve or by some transduction mechanism (such as a pain receptor on the skin). Depolarization is triggered by small local cation changes (from the adjacent membrane) on both sides of the membrane that cause the opening, initially, of sodium channel proteins. Although not many channel proteins open (at first), each opening triggers the additional opening of more channels and each open channel allows sodium ions to enter the cell at the rate of 4000 per msec. Therefore, for each $\mu m^2$ of membrane, there is an influx of some 32,000 sodium ions for the 200-$\mu$sec period when the peak of depolarization is maximal between $+10$ and $+22$ mV. This represents the action potential. It is important to realize, then, that the opening (as well as the closing) of the channel proteins is sensitive to the local concentration of adjacent cations. As the sodium ion channel proteins open, the potassium ion channel proteins also begin to open, but at a significantly slower rate, and potassium

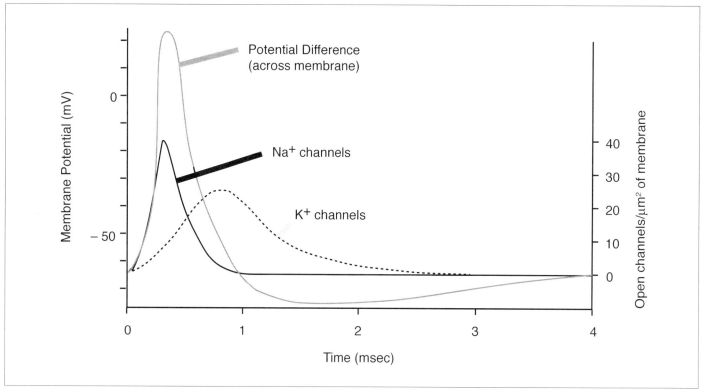

**FIGURE 7-1   Graphic representation of an action potential and ion transport at a point along a nerve axon.**

At time zero depolarization from adjacent tissue reaches the point represented. Within 0.5 msec all the sodium channel proteins (*black line*) have opened and the potassium channel proteins (*dotted line*) begin to open. In this period, the negative potential drops, as sodium ions pour into the cell, so that the potential difference actually becomes positive and remains so until 0.6 msec has elapsed. However, the exiting of potassium ions (which reaches a maximum at ∼0.9 msec) causes the potential to drop back to—and past—its original value. Recovery to the original potential is delayed until 4 msec has elapsed. During the recovery period, additional action potentials cannot take place. (Adapted from Hodgkin, 1976.)

ions begin to leave the cell. This action of potassium ions then causes sodium ion channel proteins to close. As the closing of sodium ion channel proteins continues, the potential voltage across the membranes decreases to a value somewhat below the resting potential (at time zero). When all the sodium ion channel proteins have closed, the potassium ion channel proteins begin to close also. The period of time during which the potential difference is lower than normal is described as being *refractory*. During this period (about 3 msec), no sodium ion channel proteins can be reopened by a succeeding wave of depolarization. This limits the rate of succeeding pulses of action potentials.

Action potentials can travel along nerves at rates between 1 and 100 meters per second (Mathews and van Holde, 1990). The higher rates are realized by the inclusion of layers of myelin lipid along a nerve axon. Myelin decreases the capacitance of an axon membrane. That is, myelinated nerves have a high potential with very little ability to leak cations to either side of the membrane. The areas of myelination have regular interruptions (nodes) of nonmyelination where the nerve membrane concentrates its channel proteins. Waves of depolarization in such nerves leap from node to node by causing local flows of sodium and potassium cations on both the inside and the outside of the nerve membranes (Figure 7-2). Depolarization takes place at the nodes. The advantage of a myelinated nerve is that local cation flow moves faster than the continual, connected depolarization of a nonmyelinated nerve. Although myelin lipids insulate the nerve membranes, the lipid composition of myelin requires no special lipid composition, in order to confer insulating properties to the myelin (Norton, 1981). It is simply that the myelin itself is wrapped around the nerve many times to impart an effective insulation.

Ion channel proteins themselves are relatively large proteins whose ability to transport ions is dependent on the relative ion concentration in the

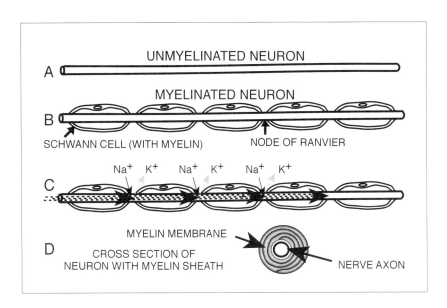

**FIGURE 7-2   Unmyelinated and myelinated nerves.**
The differences between an unmyelinated nerve (*A*) and a myelinated nerve (*B*) are the presence of myelin insulation (provided by Schwann cells) and the restriction of ion-gated channel proteins to regions between myelin sheaths known as *nodes of Ranvier*. The action potential of myelinated nerves (*C*) involves the entrance of sodium and the exiting of potassium just at the nodes. In this way depolarization leaps from node to node since depolarization cannot redevelop along the myelinated (insulated) portions of the nerve until the depolarizing wave has passed. The myelin membrane itself (shown in cross section at *D*) is wrapped around the nerve axon numerous times.

vicinity of the nerve plasma membrane. That is, the gating (opening and closing) of the channel is controlled by the cations themselves. A sodium channel protein from rat brain, for example, has a molecular weight of 320 kd (Catterall et al., 1990). It consists of three glycoprotein chains ($\alpha$, 260 kd; $\beta_1$, 36 kd; and $\beta 2$, 33 kd. Sodium ions enter neurons through a channel (pore) in the $\alpha$-chain (Figure 7-3a). One of the transmembrane segments of the $\alpha$-chain (S-4) has been designated as the voltage-sensitive (cation-sensitive) region that opens the pore.

When an action potential reaches the terminal region of an axon, where the synaptic cleft is located, it opens a channel protein specific for calcium ions rather than sodium ions. This channel is also sensitive to the local cation concentration (see Figure 7-3B for a general diagram of a neural synapse). The inflow of calcium ions brings about the fusion of vesicles in the cytoplasm with the presynaptic membrane and the subsequent release of the vesicle contents, which are neurotransmitters. The neurotransmitters diffuse across the narrow space of the synaptic cleft ($\sim$ 20 nm or 200 Å) and bind briefly to receptors on the postsynaptic membrane. Activation, through binding, of the receptors causes a postsynaptic response (both

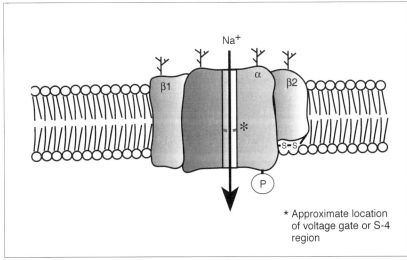

**FIGURE 7-3   (A) Ion or voltage-gated ion channel protein for sodium ions.**
The $\alpha$-polypeptide provides the energy (phosphate group), the channel, and the gate (S-4 region) for ion transport. The S-4 region is sensitive to the local concentration of cations, such that a decrease in negative potential (i.e., increase in cation concentration) triggers its opening. (Adapted from Catterall et al, 1990.) Figure is continued on the next page.

A

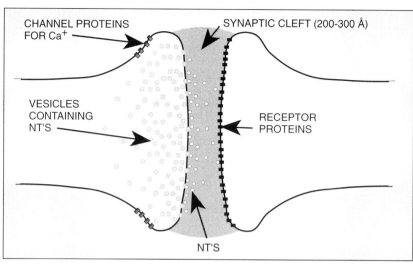

**FIGURE 7-3  (B) Diagram of a typical synaptic cleft.**
When a wave of depolarization arrives in the synaptic region, channel proteins for calcium open and calcium ions enter the presynaptic nerve. This causes vesicles containing neurotransmitters (NTs) to fuse to the presynaptic membrane facing the cleft. Upon fusion, the vesicles release their NT bundle into the cleft, where the NTs diffuse to the postsynaptic membrane and bind to receptor proteins. The binding activates a particular postsynaptic biochemical event, resulting in an excitatory post synaptic potential (EPSP) or an inhibitory postsynaptic potential (IPSP).

biochemical and physiological) that operates by a mechanism often similar to the action of hormones (see Chapter 6). The response, as previously noted, may consist of depolarization or hyperpolarization of postsynaptic neurons or contraction of muscle tissue. The biochemistry of these responses has been already partially described and is detailed further on.

## Review of Neurotransmitters and Receptor Proteins (Including Ocular Autonomic Functions)

Neurotransmitters fall into four chemical classes: acetylcholine, catecholamines, amino acids, and amino acid derivatives (Table 7-1, Figure 7-4). Some peptides have also been described as neurotransmitters that might better be labeled *neuromodulators*. A neuromodulator (neurohormone) is regarded by some as a compound with neurotransmitter properties for which experimental evidence of neurotransmission is incomplete. Others refer to them as molecules that modulate or "fine tune" the responses of neurotransmitters at the same synaptic cleft. Examples of neuromodulators are neurotensin and the enkephalins.

**TABLE 7-1   Some Neurotransmitters and Their Properties**

| Class | Example | Postsynaptic Response | Locations/ Characteristics |
|---|---|---|---|
| Acetylcholine | Acetylcholine | E/I | PNS, ANS. Fast nicotinic response, slow muscarinic response |
| Catecholamine | Norepinephrine* | E/I | CNS, ANS, retina |
| | Dopamine | I | CNS, retina |
| Amino acid | Glutamic acid* | E | CNS, retina |
| | Glycine | I | Spinal cord, retina |
| Amino acid derivative | Serotonin | I | CNS, retina |
| | γ-Aminobutyric acid | I | CNS, retina |

Key: PNS, peripheral nervous system; ANS, autonomic nervous system; CNS, central nervous system; E, excitatory; I, inhibitory.

*Epinephrine and aspartic acid may also act as neurotransmitters.

**FIGURE 7-4   The molecular structures of three neurotransmitters (acetylcholine, γ-aminobutyric acid, and norepinephrine) and one neuromodulator, met-enkephalin.**

Most investigators now consider neuromodulators to be capable of increasing or decreasing the effect produced by a neurotransmitter at a specific synaptic cleft. Their effects are similar to, although much weaker than, those produced by pain killers and mood-altering substances. They have their own receptor proteins.

Acetylcholine has been the most heavily investigated of all neurotransmitters. It is synthesized in the terminal axon bulb from acetyl CoA (see Chapter 3) and choline (an essential dietary component) by the enzyme choline acetyltransferase. When synthesized, it is incorporated into terminal vesicles. After acetylcholine has been released from its vesicle into the synaptic cleft and bound to its postsynaptic receptor protein, it is inactivated by hydrolysis with the enzyme acetylcholinesterase. The enzyme is located within the synaptic cleft. Inactivation is necessary to prevent excessive stimulation of the receptor proteins. The metabolism of acetylcholine is shown in Figure 7-5. Acetylcholinesterase is a very fast catalyst. Its turnover number of 25,000 molecules per second may be compared with that of lactate dehydrogenase (see Chapter 2), which catalyzes only 1000 molecules per second (Stryer, 1988). Clinically, the esterase is important since it can be inhibited by agents such as physostigmine to produce a controlled, temporary increase in the amount of acetylcholine available to stimulate receptor proteins. In the ocular autonomic nervous system, physostigmine has been useful in lowering the intraocular pressure of glaucoma patients. Other, more powerful agents have been used to totally inhibit the enzyme, such as insect sprays (e.g., parathion) and nerve gases (e.g., sarin) (Figure 7-6).

Receptor proteins for acetylcholine consist of two different membrane proteins, the *nicotinic receptor protein* and the *muscarinic receptor protein*. The nicotinic receptor (molecular weight 282 kd [Mathews and van Holde,

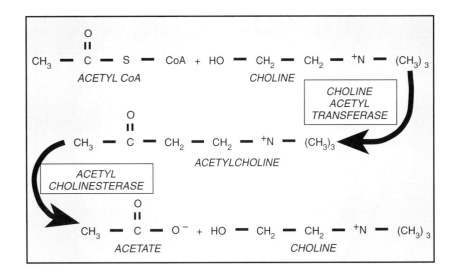

**FIGURE 7-5   Synthesis and degradation of acetylcholine.**

Synthesis occurs in the presynaptic neuron, whereas degradation occurs in the synaptic cleft.

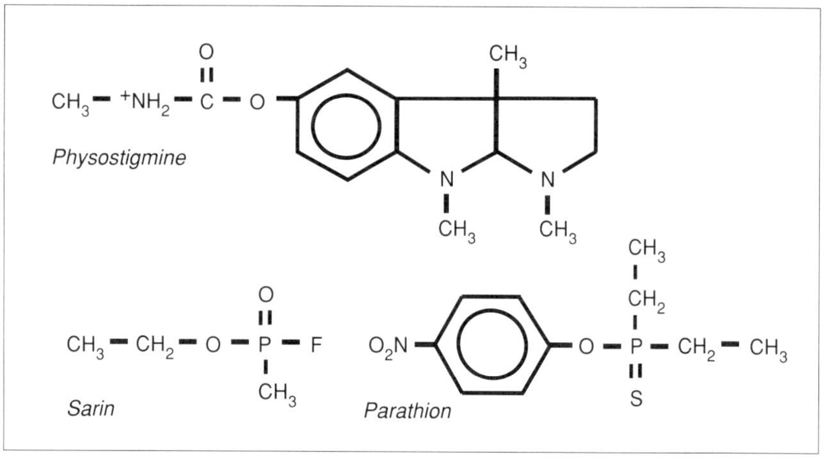

**FIGURE 7-6   Three inhibitors of acetylcholinesterase.**
Physostigmine is an alkaloid (a basic organic compound
that contains nitrogen). It was first found in Colobar beans
(from an African climbing plant). Its inhibition is temporary
and controllable. It is used as a pharmaceutical agent. Sarin
is a dangerous neurotoxin that completely inhibits
acetylcholineesterase by covalently binding to its active
site, where it forms a phosphate ester. Parathion, a much
less toxic variant of sarin, is used as an insecticide. The
phosphoryl containing inhibitors cause their destructive
events by bringing on respiratory paralysis.

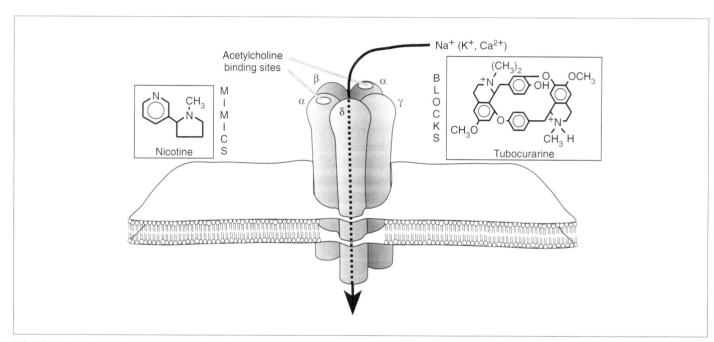

**FIGURE 7-7   The receptor for acetylcholine.**
This protein is a channel protein for sodium
predominately, though some potassium and calcium ions
may pass through. It is gated (opened) by acetylcholine
rather than by local changes in cation concentration.
Tubocurarine blocks the acetylcholine-binding sites. The
Greek letters label the different polypeptide chains that
constitute the molecule, here shown imbedded in its
plasma membrane. (Adapted from Kandel and Siegelbaum,
1991.)

1990]) is somewhat similar to the sodium channel protein in size and function. However, this channel protein is not opened by a change in cation
concentration, but by having a neurotransmitter bind to it. It is composed of
five glycoprotein subunits that, together, form a pore for cation transport. It
is named after the natural substance nicotine, which can also bind to it and
stimulate the opening of its channel. Substances that imitate neurotransmitters are known as *agonists* (Greek: *agōnistēs*, competitors). On the other
hand, curare (tubocurarine, a well-known neurotoxin) binds to and blocks
the receptor. Substances that block (prevent) receptor function are known
as *antagonists*. The nicotine receptor molecule is shown in Figure 7-7. Synaptic junctions that use nicotinic receptor proteins are considered fast
(about 1 msec) and are commonly found between nerve axons and muscles
in the peripheral nervous system and between ganglionic synapses of the
autonomic nervous system. In the autonomic nervous system this would
include parasympathetic and sympathetic activity of the iris and ciliary
body muscles in the eye. In effect, pupil size and lens focus are controlled by
the use of these receptor proteins.

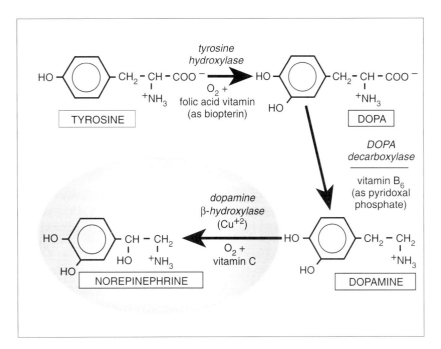

**FIGURE 7-8    The synthesis of norepinephrine.**
Three enzymes complete the process from tyrosine.
Norepinephrine is a feedback inhibitor of tyrosine
hydroxylase. This limits the synthetic rate of
norepinephrine. Note the vitamin requirements in each
step. The final stage (*in gray oval*) takes place in the
presynaptic vesicles, whereas the preceding stages occur in
the presynaptic cytoplasm. Norepinephrine is
preferentially conserved after use by reuptake (transport)
to the presynaptic neuron.

Muscarinic receptor proteins, by contrast, are considered slow receptors.
That is, the receptor, instead of directly opening a cation channel, activates
a G protein (see Chapter 6 and Figure 6-5) whose action may ultimately
cause any of the following biochemical events: stimulation of potassium
channel proteins, inhibition of adenylate cyclase, stimulation of phospholipase C, and modulation of the activity of phospholipase $A_2$ (Hulme et al.,
1991). In this sense, muscarinic receptor proteins are more like hormone
receptor proteins. The end effect of these changes in enzyme activity is to
increase or decrease potassium ion transport, decrease calcium ion transport, or increase general cation transport (Nicoll et al., 1990) in the postsynaptic cell. These events occur over a period of 100 msec and may be much
longer (MacIntosh, 1981). Although the actual structure of the receptor has
not been described, it is thought to resemble most G protein receptors, in
which a single polypeptide passes through the plasma membrane seven
times in the form of an $\alpha$-helix (see, for example, the rhodopsin molecule,
Figure 1-16). Muscarinic receptors occur in all the effector cells (smooth
muscles) stimulated by the parasympathetic nervous system. In the eye,
only pupillary and ciliary constriction are affected to, respectively, decrease
light intake and focus on near objects.

The effector cells of the sympathetic system are stimulated by norepinephrine and have one or more of its receptor proteins on their postsynaptic membrane. The neurotransmitter norepinephrine (NE, Figure 7-4) is
derived from the amino acid tyrosine (Coyle and Snyder, 1981). Three enzymes are required for its synthesis as well as molecular oxygen, three
vitamins, and copper (cupric) ions. The complete synthesis takes place in
the presynaptic region of the neuron that releases NE. However, the synthetic pathway is compartmentalized or divided between the cytoplasm
and the vesicles that store NE (Figure 7-8). Norepinephrine is predominately conserved, after binding to its receptor, by an active transport process (reuptake mechanism). This process, involving a transport protein and
Na, K-ATPase, moves the neurotransmitter back into the presynaptic cytoplasm (Coyle and Snyder, 1981), where it is taken up again into presynaptic

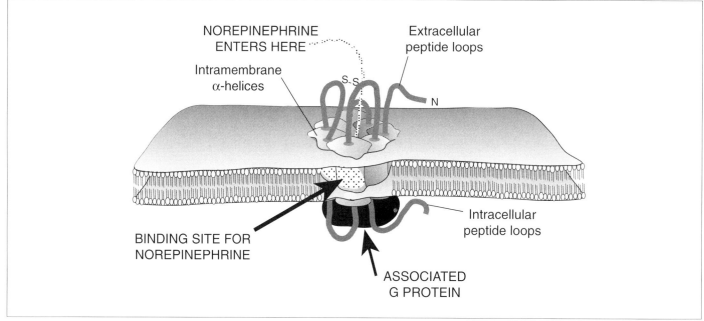

NOREPINEPHRINE ENTERS HERE

Extracellular peptide loops

Intramembrane α-helices

S-S

N

BINDING SITE FOR NOREPINEPHRINE

Intracellular peptide loops

ASSOCIATED G PROTEIN

**FIGURE 7-9   Receptor protein for norepinephrine.**
The neurotransmitter binds to its receptor deep within the plasma membrane region of the receptor α-helices. Like rhodopsin and other hormone receptor proteins, this receptor is associated with a G protein that the receptor activates. Such receptor proteins have seven α-helices traversing the cell membrane. (Adapted from Harrison et al, 1991.)

vesicles. A smaller amount of the neurotransmitter is lost from the synaptic cleft and broken down enzymatically. There are four receptor proteins for NE that are designated $\alpha_1$, $\alpha_2$, $\beta_1$, and $\beta_2$.

These proteins may be further subdivided within the α-classes (Harrison et al., 1991). The apparent reasons for the existence of so many norepinephrine and epinephrine receptors are (1) their anatomical location; (2) the option for stimulation or inhibition; and (3) the need for a variety of sensitivities to neurotransmitter binding. These receptors are all found on the postsynaptic membrane except the $\alpha_2$-types, which occur on the presynaptic membrane (Weiner, 1985). All the catecholamine receptors have a general structure similar to that of $\beta_2$ receptors (Figure 7-9). The proteins characteristically have seven α-helices that pass through the membrane and a binding site deep in the plasma membrane portion of the protein, and they function by activating a G protein. They are similar to the structure of rhodopsin and other hormone receptor molecules (see Figure 1-16) that use G proteins (see Figure 6-5). It is interesting that norepinephrine and epinephrine use the same class of receptor proteins in both hormonal and neurotransmission modes. Norepinephrine has wider use as a neurotransmitter, whereas epinephrine is used more often as a hormone. In both cases the G protein associated with the receptor either stimulates adenyl cyclase (with $\beta_1$ and $\beta_2$ receptors), or inhibits (with $\alpha_2$ receptors) (see Figure 6-5). The postsynaptic muscle response parallels the stimulation or inhibition of cAMP production. Receptors that constitute the $\alpha_1$ type, however, cause stimulation of muscle response by using calcium ions as a second messenger instead of cyclic nucleotides (Martin et al., 1985; Kandel et al., 1991). The responses produced by the catecholamines are relatively slow and correspond to the responses produced by muscarinic receptors for acetylcholine. Table 7-2 shows the receptors and mechanisms used by acetylcholine and norepinephrine.

The autonomic nervous system makes extensive use of acetylcholine and norepinephrine. In the anterior segment of the eye, this system is responsible for pupil diameter, accommodation (distance focusing), modulation of intraocular pressure, and the production of tears (Figure 7-10).

**TABLE 7-2    Receptors and Mechanisms Used by Acetylcholine and Norepinephrine**

| Neurotransmitter | Receptor | Mechanism |
|---|---|---|
| Acetylcholine | Nicotinic | Fast; causes postsynaptic depolarization primarily by acting as a gate for sodium ions |
|  | Muscarinic | Slow; G protein linked either by way of cAMP or calcium ions |
| Norepinephrine | $\alpha_1$ | Slow; G protein linked through inhibition of cAMP synthesis |
|  | $\alpha_2$ | Slow; G protein linked through use of calcium ions |
|  | $\beta_1$ $\beta_2$ | Slow; G protein linked through stimulation of cAMP synthesis |

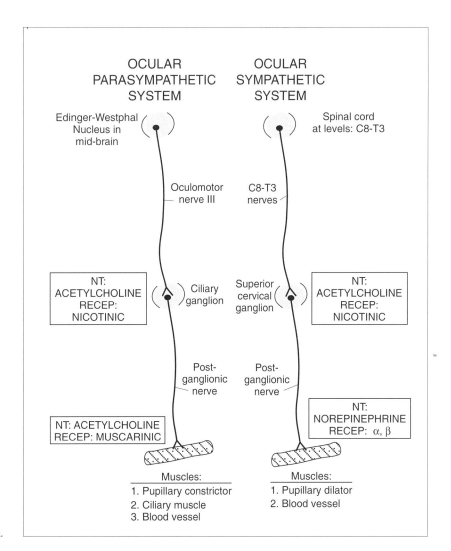

**FIGURE 7-10   Basic anatomical and neurochemical properties of ocular autonomic nerves.**
These nerves also supply innervation for tear production, especially the parasympathetic division, and eyelid tension. Note the difference in neurotransmitters and receptors in the terminal nerves of each division. RECEP = receptor protein.

## Neurochemistry of the Retina

The transduction of light in the retina was discussed previously (Chapter 6, Figures 6-7, 6-8, 6-9). However, in order to understand how the light signal is transferred to area 17 of the brain biochemically, some knowledge of the anatomical and physiological characteristics of the retina is needed. Figure 7-11

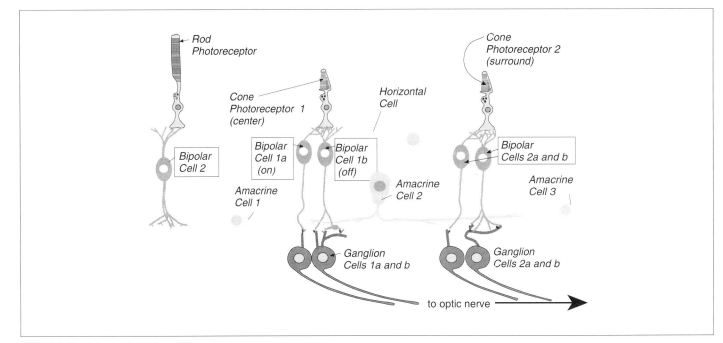

**FIGURE 7-11    Schematic outline of the principal neurons of the retina.**

Though most neurons are connected by classical synaptic junctions using neurotransmitters, some facilitate direct chemical ion transfer by use of gap junctions. These include rod-to-rod, rod-to-cone, and cone-to-cone connections (not shown). Also not shown are interplexiform cells and the glial cells of Müller. The former transfer signals from amacrine cells to horizontal cells. The latter act as cell insulators, retina boundaries, and maintenance cells for photoreceptors. See text for other cell functions. (Adapted from Tessier-Lavigne, 1991.)

shows a simplified scheme of most of the functional neurons in a mammalian retina. The most direct route of a light signal (on-center mechanism) would proceed from a cone photoreceptor onto a bipolar cell and then onto a ganglion cell. From the ganglion cell, the signal leaves the retina and proceeds to the lateral geniculate nucleus, where nerves (optic radiation fibers) leaving that nucleus send their processes to the primary visual cortex of area 17. Such a pathway, for the retina only, is shown in Figure 7-12. The pathway proceeds from the cone photoreceptor via synapse 1 (all synapses are circled) to bipolar cell 1a and on to the ganglion cell by way of synapse 2. The neurotransmitter of synapse 1 (and of all rod and cone photoreceptors) is considered to be *glutamate* (glutamic acid), although aspartate (aspartic acid) may be present in smaller amounts (Ehinger and Dowling, 1987). In the dark, or in dark-adapted conditions, both photoreceptor types continuously release their neurotransmitters to receptors on bipolar cells. This is rather unusual, since nerves generally release little or no neurotransmitter when they are inactive. This situation, however, is the direct result of the continuous flow of sodium ions known as *the dark current*, through the photoreceptors (see Figures 6-8, 6-9). When the sodium ion flow is interrupted by light transduction, the resulting hyperpolarization (i.e., build-up of net negative charge) in the photoreceptors decreases the release of glutamate. The resulting decrease in glutamate reception causes cation channel proteins for sodium to open in the bipolar postsynaptic membrane. This, in turn, brings about the release of bipolar neurotransmitter to ganglion cell receptors at synapse 2 (Tessier-Lavigne, 1991). The specific neurotransmitter for the ON signal in the bipolar cell has not yet been identified. The OFF signal, which occurs when light is turned off or suddenly decreased, proceeds by synapse 1 to bipolar cell 1b (see Figure 7-12). However, the receptor in this bipolar cell imitates the action of rhodopsin by *closing* channel proteins for sodium using a cGMP mechanism (see Figures 6-7, 6-8). As a result of this, the bipolar cell hyperpolarizes and decreases its release of glutamate to its ganglion cell at synapse 3. This action activates the

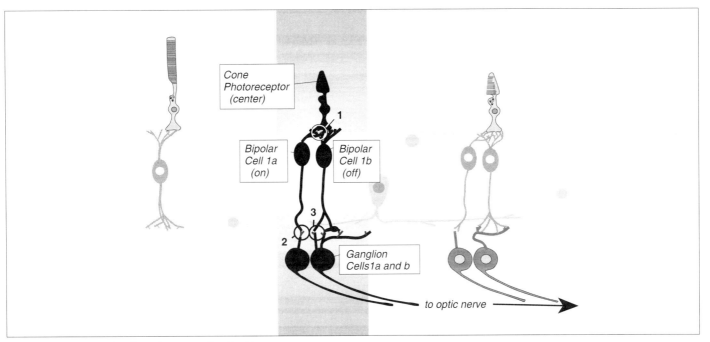

**FIGURE 7-12   Principal cells and synapses involved in cone center *on* and *off* light reception.**
The area that is involved is outlined in gray. Signals are sent through blackened cells. (Adapted from Tessier-Lavigne, 1991.)

ganglion cell (1b in the figure) in the same manner that hyperpolarization of a photoreceptor activates bipolar cell 1a.

Indirect activation mechanisms or partial inhibition of activated ganglion cells are controlled by so-called surround physiology, which involves light signals received by other cone photoreceptors nearby. One purpose of an indirect mechanism is to enhance visual acuity, the ability to distinguish borders or edges of an object. When a greater amount of light is detected by an adjacent (or surround) cone photoreceptor, the synapse sends the signal in two directions (Figure 7-13). The most direct route is to bipolar cell 2a. The signal produces the same action as the cone photoreceptor in Figure 7-12 using the same neurotransmitters and receptors. In addition, the inhibition of glutamate release from a surround cone photoreceptor activates a horizontal cell that will release γ-aminobutyric acid (GABA) as a neurotransmitter onto a center cone photoreceptor. The receptor protein, whose characteristics are unknown, continues the normal release of glutamate from the center cone photoreceptor (as though a normal dark current existed) and, therefore, *prevents* release of neurotransmitter from bipolar cell 1a (*on*). In other words, it turns off what should have been a signal from the center cone photoreceptor (Ehinger and Dowling, 1987; Berson, 1992; Tessier-Lavigne, 1991).

Rod photoreceptors, whose physiology is more concerned with detection of low levels of light, are indirectly connected to ganglion cells by way of amacrine cell synapses (Figure 7-14). The sequence of connections is this: rod photoreceptor to rod bipolar cell (synapse 1), using glutamate as a neurotransmitter; rod bipolar cell to amacrine cell (synapse 2), using an unknown neurotransmitter; amacrine cell to cone bipolar cell (on synapse 3), possibly using indoleamine as a neurotransmitter (see Ehinger and Dowling, 1987) and, finally, cone bipolar cell to ganglion cell (synapse 4), using an unknown neurotransmitter. These pathways, transmitters, and receptors are summarized in Table 7-3. Much of the information concerning synapses and neuroransmitters in the retina was obtained only recently. Some is still

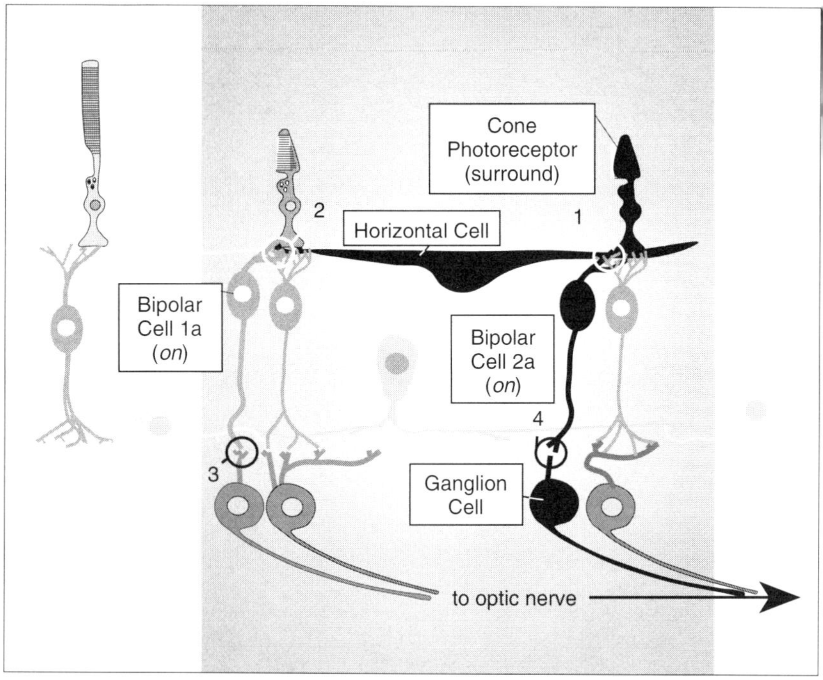

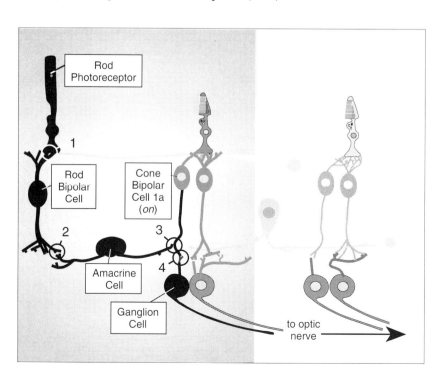

**FIGURE 7-13   Principal cells and synapses involved in cone surround *on* light reception.**
The area involved is outlined in gray. Signals are sent through blackened cells. (Adapted from Tessier-Lavigne, 1991.)

being gathered. For these reasons, it is not yet possible to construct a completely meaningful story of retinal function and disease in relation to the neurochemistry of this tissue.

## Ocular Neurochemical Pathology

In general, neurotransmission in the eye functions well, except when it is disrupted by degenerative conditions (such as retinitis pigmentosa or by nerve lesions outside the eye such as those associated with Horner's syndrome). Recently, Harnois and Dipaola (1990) have found a correlation

**FIGURE 7-14   Principal cells and synapses involved in rod light reception.**
The area concerned is outlined in gray. Signals are sent through blackened cells. Note that there is no direct connection between rod bipolar cells and ganglion cells. (Adapted from Tessier-Lavigne, 1991.)

**ABLE 7-3    Some Synaptic Pathways of the Retina**

| Type | Synapse (Neurotransmitter) | Receptor Mechanism |
|---|---|---|
| Cone, *center, on* | Photoreceptor → bipolar (glutamate) | Opening of sodium ion channel proteins |
| | Bipolar → ganglion (unknown) | Unknown |
| Cone, *center, off* | Photoreceptor → bipolar (glutamate) | Closing of sodium ion channel proteins |
| | Bipolar → ganglion (glutamate) | Opening of sodium ion channel proteins |
| Cone, *surround, on* | Photoreceptor* → horizontal (glutamate) | Opening of sodium ion channel proteins |
| | Horizontal → photoreceptor (γ-aminobutyric acid) | Maintenance of glutamate release |
| | Photoreceptor[†] → bipolar (glutamate) | Opening of sodium ion channel proteins |
| | Bipolar → ganglion (unknown) | Unknown |
| Rod, low light | Photoreceptor → rod bipolar (glutamate) | Closing of sodium ion channel proteins |
| | Rod bipolar → amacrine (unknown) | Opening of sodium ion channel proteins |
| | Amacrine → cone bipolar (indoleamine?) | Opening of sodium ion channel proteins |

*This is the indirect pathway to the adjacent cone photoreceptor.

[†]This is the direct pathway to the ganglion cell, which is similar to the cone, center, ON type, above.

between retina levels of dopamine and visual disturbances in patients with Parkinson's disease. These patients lose some of their contrast sensitivity. Compared to normal subjects, whose average retina concentration is 1 ng dopamine per milligram of protein, untreated Parkinsonian patients were found to have levels of approximately 0.52 ng dopamine per milligram of protein. Dopamine is a neurotransmitter found in some amacrine cells. Although its function was not described in any of the previous discussion, evidence indicates that amacrine cells (some of which use dopamine) serve as intermediate cells for the lateral transfer of signals across the retina. In short, they appear to be part of an auxiliary system for visual acuity. Still another retina cell type, known as an *interplexiform cell*, may also use dopamine and may have a similar function (Ehinger and Dowling, 1987).

## Summary

Neural transmission occurs with the depolarization of nerve plasma membranes. The transmission results with the entry of sodium ions into the neuron and ceases with the sequential loss of potassium ions to the outside of the nerve. This activity is controlled by cation-gated channel proteins and is initiated by an incipient, local depolarization. In myelinated proteins ion movement is limited to nerve nodes, so that ion movement causes depolarization to leap from node to node. This increases the transmission rate greatly. At nerve synapses, neurotransmitters are released to diffuse across a small space (cleft) to bind to receptor proteins. This produces either depolarization in the postsynaptic cell and in some cells imitates the mechanism of hormones in which G proteins are intermediates that produce a physiological response. There are four classes of neurotransmitters: acetylcholine, catecholamines, amino acids, and amino acid derivatives. Of these, acetylcholine and norepinephrine have been very well described.

Acetylcholineesterase is used to degrade acetylcholine in the synapse, and inhibitors of this esterase have been used as therapeutic agents to prolong the concentration of acetylcholine in synapses where they occur.

In the eye, they have been used to control glaucoma and to restore normal pupil size after an eye examination. The two ocular autonomic systems use acetylcholine as a neurotransmitter at their ganglia. Nicotinic acetylcholine receptors are present there and produce a "fast" response. In the ocular parasympathetic division of postganglionic nerves, acetylcholine is also the neurotransmitter, but a "slower-acting" muscarinic receptor protein is found on the muscle receptor membranes. These receptors use G proteins. In the ocular sympathetic division of postganglionic nerves, norepinephrine is the neurotransmitter. Four kinds of receptor proteins are present there: $\alpha_1$, $\alpha_2$, $\beta_1$, and $\beta_2$. All are slow "acting" and make use of G proteins.

In the retina, a variety of neurotransmitters may be found. However, photoreceptor cells, some ganglion cells, and a few others that use glutamate possess an unusual mechanism by which they transmit signals. These cells normally release glutamate when they are inactive. When they detect light or a photoreceptor signal they hyperpolarize and decrease their release of glutamate. Their postsynaptic cells are themselves either hyperpolarized or depolarized, depending on their receptor mechanisms. There are several ways in which the retina responds to light and brings about a cascade of neurotransmission in amplified, inhibited, or modulated fashion: cone *on-off,* cone *center-surround,* and rod-dominated mechanisms. Each system uses a specific sequence of neurotransmitters and receptors that operate on a variety of cells.

## References

Berson EL. Electrical phenomena in the retina. *In* Hart WM (ed). *Adler's Physiology of the Eye,* 9th ed. St Louis: CV Mosby, 1992;689–690.

Catterall WA, Nunoki K, Lai Y, DeJongh K, Thomsen W, and Rossie S. Structure and modulation of voltage-sensitive sodium and calcium channels. *In* Nishizuka Y et al. (eds). *The Biology and Medicine of Signal Transduction.* New York: Raven Press, 1990;30–35.

Coyle JT, and Snyder SH. Catecholamines. *In* Siegel GJ, Albers RW, Agranoff BW, and Katzman R (eds). *Basic Neurochemistry.* New York: Little, Brown, 1981;209–210.

Ehinger B, and Dowling JE. Retinal neurocircuitry and transmission. *In* Björklund A, Hökfelt T, and Swanson LW (eds). *Handbook of Chemical Neuroanatomy,* vol 5. New York, Elsevier, 1987;389–446.

Harnois C, and DiPaola T. Decreased dopamine in the retina of patients with Parkinson's disease. *Invest Ophthalmol Vis Sci* 1990;31:2473–2475.

Harrison JK, Pearson WR, and Lynch KR. Molecular characterization of $\alpha_1$- and $\alpha_2$- adrenoceptors. *Trends Pharmacol Sci* 1991;12:62–67.

Hille B. Excitability and ionic channels. *In* Siegel GJ, Albers RW, Agranoff BW, and Katzman R (eds). *Basic Neurochemistry.* New York: Little Brown, 1981;75–106.

Hodgkin AL. Chance and design in electrophysiology: An informal account of certain experiments on nerves carried out between 1934 and 1952. *J Physiol* (London) 1976;263:1–21.

Hulme EC, Kurtenbach E, and Curtis CAM. Muscarinic acetylcholine receptors: Structure and function. *Biochemical Soc Trans* 1991;19:133–137.

Kandel ER, Schwartz JH, and Jessell TM. Synaptic transmission mediated by second messengers. *Principles of Neural Science* (3rd ed). New York: Elsevier, 1991;179–181.

Kandel ER, and Siegelbaum SA. Directly gated transmission at the nerve muscle synapse. *In* Kandel ER, Schwartz JH, and Jessell TM (eds). *Principles of Neural Science* (3rd ed). New York: Elsevier 1991;146–148.

MacIntosh FC. Acetylcholine. *In* Siegel GJ, Albers RW, Agranoff BW, and Katzman R (eds). *Basic Neurochemistry.* New York: Little, Brown, 1981;189.

Martin DW, Mayes PA, Rodwell VW, and Graimer DK. *Harper's Reivew of Biochemistry*, 20th ed. Los Altos, Calif: Lange, 1985;567–568.

Mathews CK, and van Holde KE. *Biochemistry*. Redwood City, Calif: Benjamin/Cummings, 1990;1035–1050.

Nicoll RA, Malenka RC, and Kauer JA. Functional comparison of neurotransmitter receptor subtypes in mammalian central nervous system. *Physiol Rev* 1990;70:513–565.

Norton WT. Formation, structure and biochemistry of myelin. *In* Siegel GJ, Albers RW, Agranoff BW, and Katzman R (eds). *Basic Neurochemistry.* New York: Little, Brown, 1981;63–92.

Slaughter MM, and Miller RF. Bipolar cells in the mudpuppy retina use an excitatory amino acid neurotransmitter. *Nature* 1983;303:537–538.

Stryer L. *Biochemistry*, (3rd ed). New York: WH Freeman, 1988;191.

Tessier-Lavigne M. Phototransduction and information processing in the retina. *In* Kandell ER, Schwartz JR, and Jessell TM (eds). *Principles of Neural Science*. New York, Elsevier, 1991;412–414.

Weiner N. Norepinephrine, epinephrine and the sympathomimetic amines. *In* Gilman AG, Goodman, LS, Rall TW, and Marad F (eds). *The Pharmacological Basis of Therapeutics*, 7th ed. New York: Macmillan, 1985;145–180.

# Chapter 8

# Immunochemistry

Immunology is a major scientific discipline that deals with the manner in which organisms defend themselves against foreign invasion. In respect to humankind, this is usually thought of in terms of bacterial and viral infections. However, any foreign substance may provoke an immune reaction. In fact, under unfortunate circumstances individuals may reject some of their own tissue in what is known as an autoimmune reaction. In the eye, immune reactions are normally limited to the region of the anterior segment. Here, the discussion focuses on immunochemistry and, in particular, on the biochemical substances *immunoglobulins* and *complement.* A short treatise on inflammation is included.

## Review of Immunoglobulins

Immunoglobulins are relatively large proteins that contain a minimum of four polypeptide chains. Their function is to bind to a foreign substance (a molecule or a portion of a molecule) in order to identify it and initiate an immunological defense. More will be said about this later. The history of the discovery of immunoglobulins goes back to 1847, when H. Bence Jones isolated parts of immunoglobulins from the urine of a patient who had high levels of urinary protein (Day, 1990). What Bence Jones had found were the lighter of the four polypeptide chains of immunoglobulins, and, subsequently, these became known as *Bence Jones proteins.* Immunoglobulins (also known as antibodies) have an overall conformation similar to the letter Y or the letter T. More complex forms are variations of these basic shapes. Figures 1-5 through 1-8 show the primary, secondary, tertiary, and quaternary structures of these proteins. At this point it is necessary to explain the conformation of immunoglobulins in greater detail. Figure 8-1 shows such a detailed rendering of immunoglobulin G (IgG). The four polypeptide chains are shown in various shades of black and gray. The heavier chains have four domains, each connected by random coil sequences; the lighter chains have just two domains apiece. Each domain is partially held together by an intrachain disulfide bond (S—S). Both heavy and light chains are associated by interchain disulfide bonds. Note that the two heavy chains are also bound to oligosaccharides.

Each domain is labeled as C (for constant) or V (for variable). The amino acid sequence in each C domain is always the same for a particular immunoglobulin, but the amino acid sequence in each V domain is determined by the antigen (foreign substance) with which the antibody must bind. The antigen-binding region is defined by the space between two variable domains, where binding takes place. For simple immunoglobulins, there are two binding regions per molecule. The hinge regions represent sequences of amino acids between C1 and C2 of the heavy chains that can twist or flex (Nisonoff, 1985; Day, 1990). In this way, the immunoglobulin molecule can twist back and forth from a Y to a T shape to bind to one or two antigenic molecules. All the domains of an immunoglobulin have specific roles in addition to the binding role of the V domain (Figure 8-2). For example, the C1 and C2 domains can bind to complement (discussed later), whereas the

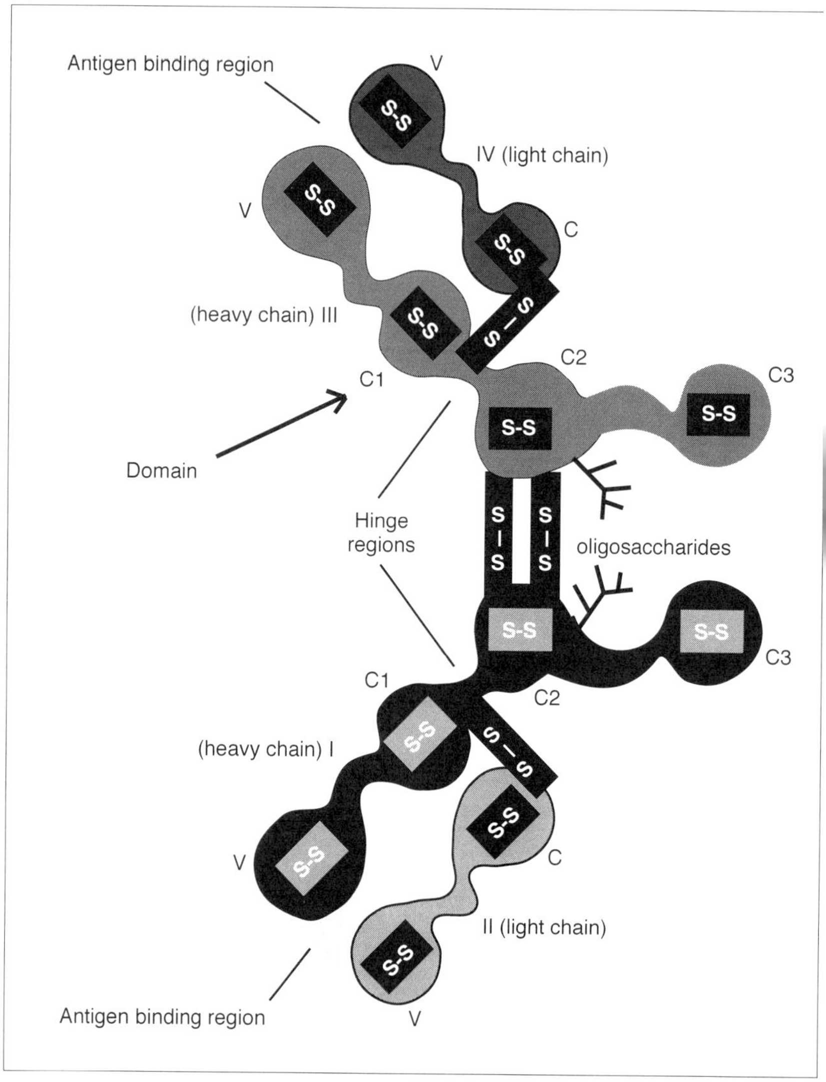

**FIGURE 8-1  A detailed diagram of immunoglobulin G.**
Shown here is subtype IgG1. The other subtypes vary in
number and position of disulfide bonds. Subtype IgG3 has
a large C2 domain on each heavy chain.

**FIGURE 8-2  The variable domain of an
immunoglobulin.**
Two classes of sequences are found here: hypervariable
(*dark shading*) and occasionally variable or conserved (*light
shading*). The hypervariable regions are specifically
synthesized to bind to one or to only a very few antigens.
The conserved sequences are synthesized primarily to
maintain the conformation of the domain and are
occasionally varied to help the hypervariable regions to
align optimally with an antigen. (Adapted from Alberts et
al., 1989b.)

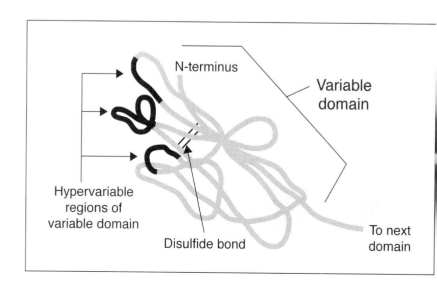

C3 domain can bind to receptor proteins on macrophages and monocytes (white blood cells). The light chain C domain, however, seems to be primarily structural in function (Roitt et al., 1985a). Three roles have been assigned to the oligosaccharides attached to immunoglobulins: (1) enhancement of water solubility, (2) protection against enzymatic degradation, and (3) facilitation in secretion from cells that produce them (Nisonoff, 1985).

There are five major classes of immunoglobulins: A, D, E, G, and M. Their characteristics are summarized in Table 8-1. Immunoglobulin A tends to form a two-molecule unit (dimer) when secreted by cells that make it. As shown in Figure 8-3, secretory IgA is joined stem-to-stem by a polypeptide called a J chain (15 kd) where J stands for "joining." Another polypeptide, termed an S chain (60 kd) where S stands for "secretory," is wrapped around the two immunoglobulin tetramer units. The S chain prevents proteolytic degradation of the immunoglobulin over and above the protection provided by the oligosaccharides. This is necessary since the precorneal tear film and other external secretions are particularly rich in degrading enzymes.

Immunoglobulin D is considered to be significant in connective tissue defense. It is not normally found in the anterior ocular fluids.

Immunoglobulin E may occur in very small quantities in the precorneal tear film, though its role is not understood. It is known that it causes release of histamine from mast cells after binding to their surface. In other parts of the body this activity is associated with the hypersensitivity reactions of asthma and hay fever as well as the eventual rejection of internal parasites (Roitt et al., 1985b).

Immunoglobulin G forms about 80% of all immunoglobulins in blood serum and is found in significant quantities in both precorneal tear film and aqueous humor. IgG is the smallest of the immunoglobulins and generally is found in interstitial fluids in largest quantities. It is even able to diffuse through the cornea itself. After a second exposure to a particular antigen, IgG is made in the greatest quantities to respond to that infection. Accordingly, IgG is considered to be the second line of defense while IgA is the first line of defense to a specific antigen. IgG can bind to surface receptor proteins of B lymphocytes in order to stimulate these cells (B-lymphocytes are

**TABLE 8-1    The Major Immunoglobulin Classes: Characteristics and Concentrations**

| Characteristic | IgA | IgD | IgE | IgG | IgM |
|---|---|---|---|---|---|
| Subclasses (No.) | 4 | None | None | 4 | None |
| Molecular weight (kd) | 160[*] | 170 | 190[†] | 146[‡] | 970[†] |
| Carbohydrate (%) | 7–11 | 10–12 | 12 | 2–3 | 9–12 |
| Primary location | Secretions | Blood vessels | Mast cells | Most tissues | Blood vessels |
| Serum [§][#](μg/mL) | 760–3900[∥] | 40 | ≪1 | 6500–15,000 | 900–3450 |
| Tear film[§][**] (μg/mL) | 1930[¶] | 0 | 0 | 4 | 18 |
| Aqueous[§][††] (μg/mL) | 10 | 0 | 0 | 70 | 0 |
| Lens[††] (μg/g) | 0 | 0 | 0 | 0 | 0 |

[*]Secretory IgA, 405 kd.
[†]H has a C4 domain on its heavy chains.
[‡]IgG3, subclass, 165 kd.
[§]Normal valve, but increases with foreign invasion.
[∥]Secretory IgA, ≤0.05 μg ml.

[¶]Value for secretory IgA; dimeric and monomeric IgA also are present.
[#]Data from Silverman et al. (1986).
[**]Data from Fullard and Tucker (1991).
[††]Data from Allansmith et al. (1973).

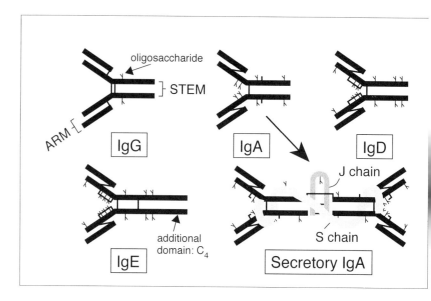

**FIGURE 8-3 Comparison of immunoglobulins A, G, D, and E.**
Note the variations and numbers of disulfide bonds (lines between chains) and oligosaccharides (y-shaped lines). IgE has an additional domain on each heavy chain with which it binds to mast cells. IgA in the precorneal tear film is principally secretory IgA. (Adapted from Roitt et al., 1985b).

the cells that synthesize immunoglobulins). Immunoglobulin G is the second most important antibody in ocular tissues. It is present in both precorneal tear film and aqueous humor.

Immunoglobulin M (Figure 8-4) is a very large molecule composed of five tetrapeptide units (a pentamer) as well as a J polypeptide (the same one found in secretory IgA). One IgM unit has 10 antigen-binding sites and is one of the first immunoglobulins made after "recognition" of an antigen, that is, after IgA binds to the antigen. IgM tends to agglutinate or form large molecular complexes of foreign bacteria. It is present in the precorneal tear film.

Central to all immunoglobulin function is the antigen-antibody reaction, which takes place between the ends of the variable domains of the heavy

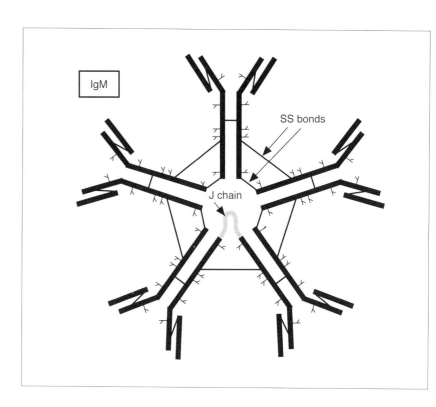

**FIGURE 8-4 The large IgM molecule.**
This conformation is suggested by some electron photomicrographs; however individual immunoglobulin units may not be in the same plane around the disulfide bond ring that connects them. (Adapted from Roitt et al., 1985b.)

**FIGURE 8-5    Schematic diagram of a radioimmunoassay.**
A radioimmunoassay combines the sensitivities of both radioactive and immunochemical reactions. In the assay, a radioactive antigen competes with a nonradioactive antigen for the possession of a binding site on an antibody. The assay measures the radioactivity on the bound antibody. Accordingly, the greater the binding of a nonradioactive antigen on an antibody, the lower the level of radioactivity measured. Since the sample (antigen) contains no radioactivity, greater amounts of sample bound to the antibody will have less radioactivity when counted by liquid scintillation (note standard curve). The control gives the reference radioactivity for 100% binding of radioactive antigen. In the assay, standard, known amounts of nonradioactive antigens are reacted in the upper row and compared with the control. From this, a standard curve is constructed (shown on right). One or more unknown samples are run. The percentages of radioactivity in the antibodies are measured (y-axis) and intersected with the standard curve to obtain the concentration of antigen (x-axis). This method, for example, is very useful in determining very low concentrations of hormones in blood.

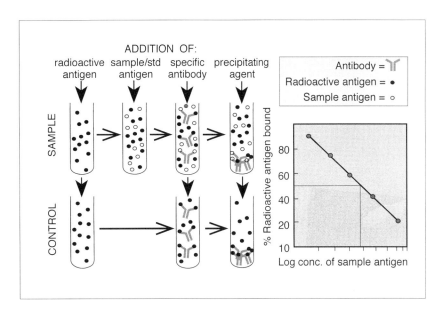

and light chains (the antibody-binding region seen in Figure 8-1). An antigen (Greek: *anti genein*, to make against) can be any substance that produces an antibody (immunoglobulin) to which it will bind. It is important to emphasize that for most antigen-antibody reactions the immunoglobulin binds to only a portion of the antigen. The portion that is bound is called an *antigenic determinant*, or *epitope*. The epitope may be a short peptide, an oligosaccharide, a lipid molecule, or even a nucleic acid fragment. This is usually the case with bacteria and viruses, in which an antibody binds to a portion of the prokaryotic surface. Besides such organisms, proteins themselves ($>1$ kd) and large polysaccharides ($>1000$ kd) may be antigenic (Bach, 1982). Some substances may become antigenic when combined with a larger carrier molecule. These substances, called *haptens* (Greek: *haptein,* to fasten), include a number of small organic chemicals. Among these are substances containing azo groups ($-N\!\!=\!\!N-$) that form colored diazonium complexes with the aromatic amino acids of their carrier proteins. These colored antigens can be used spectrophotometrically to determine the number of haptens when studying antigen-antibody reactions. Such assays were a precursor to the extremely sensitive radioimmunoassays that were later developed by Berson and Yalow (1968). In radioimmunoassays (Figure 8-5), antigen-antibody reactions are coupled to radioactive compounds to give extremely sensitive assays (to $10^{-15}$ M) for hormones and other substances present in very low concentrations in tissues.

The nature of the antigen-antibody reaction is complex and involves all of the noncovalent forces described under protein structure formation (Chapter 1) as well as the correct conformational requirements, as needed, for example, between enzyme and substrate (Chapter 2). For review and reinforcement, these factors are given in Table 8-2. It is emphasized that the antigen-antibody reaction is the sum of all these factors. Naturally, some substances produce better reactions than others. Just like substrate-enzyme binding, each antibody is specific for only one or a few antigens. The kinetics of binding are similar, therefore, to the kinetics of substrate-enzyme affinity.

**TABLE 8-2    Factors That Contribute to Antigen-Antibody Reactions at the Antigen-Binding Region of an Immunoglobulin**

| Factor | Type | Characteristic |
|---|---|---|
| Chemical bond | Hydrogen | Sharing of a hydrogen atom due to partial charges between two atoms |
| | Electrostatic | Full positive and/or negative charge(s) on antigen and/or antibody, respectively |
| | van der Waals | Induced partial charge between two atoms (not involving hydrogen) |
| Nonpolar bond | Hydrophobic | Association of molecules away from a water (polar) environment |
| Conformation | Lock and key | Complementary shape of antigen and hypervariable part of V domain |

Genetically, it is of great interest to understand how an antigen (or antigenic determinant) can specify the synthesis of immunoglobulins that bind to one or a very few, similar antigens. Currently, this process is only partially understood. B cells or B lymphocytes are the site of immunoglobulin synthesis. In the adult human, B cells are initially formed in the bone marrow and then transported to lymphoid tissues prior to full development as B plasma cells. When they leave the bone marrow they can only produce IgM and IgD which bind to the cell surface membrane at the stem side of the molecule (Banchereau and Rousset, 1992). In the lymphoid tissues, the B cells are induced to make specific immunoglobulins belonging to the other classes. This they do by binding antigens to the nonspecific IgD and IgM that is already attached to the B plasma cell's membrane surface (Figure 8-6). The synthesis of immunoglobulins by these developing B cells, however, actually begins in the bone marrow, when the cells become "committed" to the synthesis of first light chains then heavy chains to produce IgM, then IgD. These immunoglobulins have hydrophobic "tails" (the tips of the stems) that bind to the membranes of the B cells. When antigens encounter IgM and IgD bound to the nascent B cells, they bind to these antibodies and transmit a signal to begin specific antibody synthesis. Such short-lived, high-output B lymphocytes are called *plasma cells*. Figure 8-7 depicts the

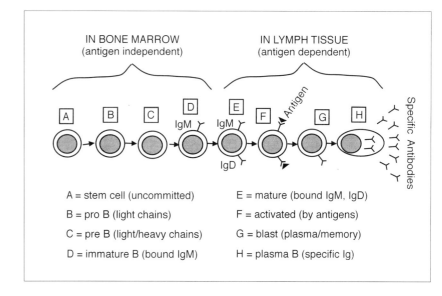

**FIGURE 8-6    The development of plasma B cells from uncommitted stem cells.**
The cells begin by making surface-bound antibodies (D and E), which induce (by antigen binding, F) the production of large quantities of specific antibodies (H). (Adapted from Banchereau and Rousset, 1992.)

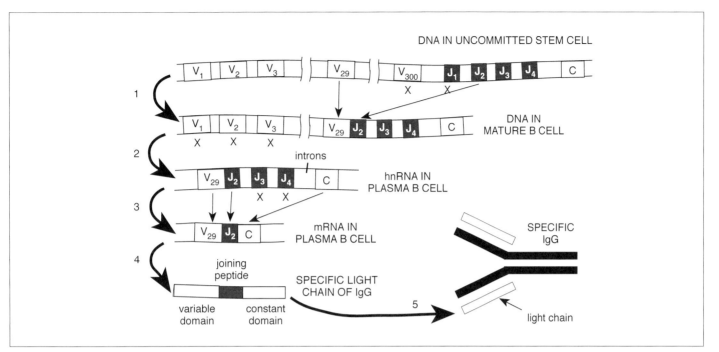

**FIGURE 8-7    The genetic component of the antibody diversity hypothesis for the production of light chains of specific antibodies.**

In the determination of a specific antibody, the cell deletes unwanted exons as in steps 1, 2, and 3. In this case exons: $V_{29}$, $J_2$, and C have been joined as mRNA. In step 4, the specific light peptide is synthesized and incorporated into IgG (step 5). See text for further explanation.

current understanding of how the selection process operates, at the genetic level, for the synthesis of so many different kinds of antibodies. This process, which represents the "antibody diversity hypothesis," is shown in the figure only for the light chains of IgG. The top diagram represents uncommitted B cells in the bone marrow (or in the fetal liver). In this case the DNA contains the codes for 300 separate sequences of the variable domain (V genes). It also contains, downstream, the codes for four separate peptides that will connect or join the V and C domains (J genes). It should be emphasized that the J genes do *not* code for the J protein in secretory IgA and IgM, but for a joining peptide between the V and C domains. Last, and still farther downstream, is the code for the constant domain (a single code known as the *C gene*). When the stem cell becomes committed to B-cell development, the DNA containing all these codes recombines by excision (cutting out) of part of the DNA. In one example, as in the next lower diagram of Figure 8-7, all of the V genes 30 through 300 have been excised and V gene 29 has been directly joined to J gene 2. J gene 1 was also excised. Even though V genes 1 through 28 are still present, they are not directly connected in sequence to the J2 gene and are, therefore, inactive. This is also true of the J3 and J4 genes. This is the form of DNA that exists in a B cell that is ready to begin IgG synthesis. In the transcription state of forming hnRNA, only V gene 29, J genes 2, 3, and 4, and the C gene are transcribed. When hnRNA is processed to mRNA, all the introns, as well as the inactive J3 and J4 exons, are spliced out of the gene sequence. This leaves the V29, J2, and C codes for the specific light chain of IgG to be translated and assembled into an IgG that will bind to a specific antigen. The processing of the heavy chains is similar but more complex. In the consideration of all the possible combinations of heavy and light chains, as well as three variations of splicing V and J genes, it may be possible for cells to make more than $10^8$ different kinds of antibodies from committed and activated B cells. This number, however, may be too large, since Zachau (1989) has reported that the number of human

V genes may only be 84 rather than 300. However, even if there were only 84 V genes, it would still be possible to make $3.4 \times 10^{7}$ antibodies!

## Ocular Immunoglobulins

As can be seen from Table 8-1, three antibodies occur in significant amounts in ocular tissues: IgA, IgG, and IgM. The IgA in the precorneal tear film is primarily the secretory type (see Figure 8-3). It is assembled from dimeric IgA in the lacrimal gland epithelial cells. These epithelial cells synthesize the S-chain polypeptide that surrounds the IgA molecules and protects them from degradation (Smolin and O'Connor, 1986). IgM is limited to the precorneal tear film due to its large size, which prevents its diffusion through tissues such as the corneal stroma. IgE has been reported to occur, but since it normally is tightly bound to mast cells, its occurrence in free form is dubious (note its low concentration in blood serum [Table 8-1]). The concentrations of ocular immunoglobulins, as given in Table 8-1, reflect normal concentrations in the healthy eye. The normal occurrence of immunoglobulins in the eye is fairly limited to the precorneal tear film, the aqueous, the ocular blood vessels, and the outermost tissues such as the cornea and the sclera. In the deeper ocular tissues such as the lens and the vitreous, no antibodies are usually found. The actual determination of immunoglobulin concentrations in tears (in both normal and disease states) has been frustrated by tear sampling techniques. This is particularly true in resting tears versus tears obtained by stimulation. In general, the more tear production is stimulated (e.g., by emotional or chemical means) the lower the content of immunoglobulin and other protein contents due to reflex dilution. The manner of collecting tears for assay of immunoglobulins is also important. Tears collected with small sponges tend to be contaminated with conjunctival secretions and tears obtained with filter paper (Schirmer strips) may be reflex stimulated (diluted tears). However, tears that are drawn into glass capillary tubes do not have these drawbacks if the collection is done carefully.

As antigens either invade the ocular surface or enter the tissue itself, the immunoglobulin concentration changes considerably. For example, when the corneal surface is exposed to an antigen such as herpes virus, IgM is the first antibody to respond from the precorneal tear film. The increase in IgM level is followed by increases in IgG and secretory IgA (Smolin and O'Connor, 1986). As the infection progresses, herpes antigens are found in the cornea, conjunctiva, tear film, iris, and trigeminal ganglion. It may be recalled from Chapter 5 that nerve ganglia are storage sites for inactive forms of this virus. In the cornea, infected cells may have some of the viral antigens incorporated into their plasma membranes. This action will trigger antigen-antibody reactions against the cells themselves. Viruses that have not yet invaded cells are also attacked by antibodies, especially by secretory IgA, which prevents the virus from attaching to uninfected cells. IgG causes phagocytosis of the antigen virus, as described in the next section. McBride and Ward (1987) were able to measure the quantities of IgG subtypes that respond to herpes simplex invasion. Their findings (Table 8-3) indicate a seven-fold increase in the subtype IgG4.

Recent work suggests that the immunoglobulins that stimulate the thyroid gland in Graves' disease (Chapter 6) also react with the extra-ocular muscle tissues (Wall, et al., 1991). This autoimmune reaction may be what causes these tissues to swell in this disease.

**TABLE 8-3   Comparison of IgG Subtypes in the Tears of Individuals with and without Herpes Infections**

| Individual | Concentration of IgG* (μg/mL tears) | |
| --- | --- | --- |
| | *IgG1* | *IgG4* |
| Control (uninfected, n = 5) | 2.01 | 0.08 |
| Herpes (infected, n = 9) | 2.22 | 0.56 |

Data from McBride and Ward (1987).

*The tears in this study are presumably stimulated when compared with the unstimulated tear data contained in Table 8-1. IgG2 and IgG3 subtypes are not found in the tears of individuals.

## Complement

Complement is a collection of related proteins, of which most are either proteolytic enzymes or membrane-binding proteins. Complement has two principal functions: (1) direct destruction of foreign organisms by membrane lysis, and (2) activation of phagocytosis (cell engulfment) following chemotaxis (cell movement induced by chemicals). Complement is, therefore, a biochemical immune mechanism that is capable of destroying gram-negative bacteria (see Chapter 2) and some parasites as well as neutralizing some viruses. These functions will be presented in detail after a discussion of the molecular properties of complement and complement activation. Complement in the classical pathway (started by antigen-antibody reactions) is constituted by 11 separate and distinct proteins (Table 8-4): C1q, C1r, C1s, C2, C3, C4, C5, C6, C7, C8, and C9. However, since more than one protein of the same type is used in complement activation, a very large number of proteins actually constitute all of the proteins involved in one activation sequence. The mechanism is a *cascade amplification* similar to that caused by cyclic nucleotides.

The sequence of complement fixation (or activation) begins with the binding of the C1 complex (one C1q, two C1s, and two C1r molecules held together by calcium ions) to the stem portion of either IgG or IgM molecules, which are themselves bound to the membrane antigens (Figure 8-8). Upon binding to the immunoglobulin, a conformational shift of the C1 complex induces autocatalytic properties in C1s and C1r. That is, the proteins cause

**TABLE 8-4   The Proteins of Complement Activated by the Classical Pathway***

| Protein | Molecular Weight (kd) | Number of Chains | Characteristics |
| --- | --- | --- | --- |
| C1q | 410 | 18 | Ig stem–binding |
| C1r | 83 | 1 | Proteolytic zymogen |
| C1s | 83 | 1 | Proteolytic zymogen |
| C2 | 110 | 1 | Proteolytic/chemotactic |
| C3 | 190 | 2 | Proteolytic/chemotactic |
| C4 | 206 | 3 | Proteolytic zymogen |
| C5 | 190 | 2 | Membrane/chemotactic |
| C6 | 95 | 1 | Membrane-binding |
| C7 | 120 | 1 | Membrane-binding |
| C8 | 163 | 3 | Membrane-binding |
| C9 | 79 | 1 | Membrane channel |

*The classical pathway requires antibodies for activation; the alternate pathway does not.

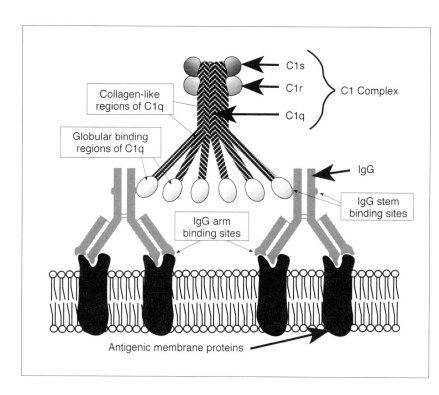

**FIGURE 8-8    The initial reactions of antibody-induced complement formation.**
When either IgG or IgM binds to the antigenic membrane proteins of an organism (such as a bacterium) C1q binds to the stem region of at least two antibodies. C1q is part of the C1 complex. Binding causes a conformational shift of the C1q molecule that is communicated to C1r and C1s. As a result, C1s becomes an esterase enzyme following activation of C1r also as an enzyme. (C1s is a substrate for C1r). No peptide chains are broken. (Adapted from Roitt et al., 1985c.)

their own activation and C1s molecules ultimately become proteolytic enzymes for the next substrate proteins in the sequence, C4 and C2 (Figure 8-9). Each C4 is broken into fragments—C4a and C4b. C4b binds to the membrane in the vicinity of the antigen-antibody complex, but C4a does not participate in the sequence. C2 is also broken into C2a and C2b fragments by C1s. C2a binds to the C4b molecule and becomes an enzyme (C3 convertase) to split C3 into C3a and C3b. The C3b fragment associates with C4b and C2b to form still another enzyme, C5 convertase. The C3a fragment has a different role, to which we shall return. C5 is split into C5a and C5b fragments. The C5b fragment binds to a nearby region of the antigen membrane and initiates the formation of a complex that contains bound C6, C7, C8, and several molecules of C9. The C9 proteins are channel-forming proteins. In order to be completely effective the C9 protein channels must eventually pierce the cytoplasmic membrane of the bacteria (Figure 8-10).

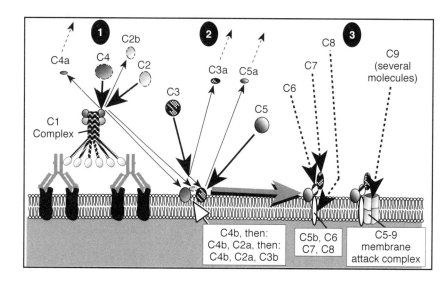

**FIGURE 8-9    The complete diagram of complement activation by the classical pathway.**
In stage 1, the C1s proteolytic enzyme is activated (Figure 8-8) to split C4 and C2. In stage 2, the activation of C3 and C5 convertase in sequence begins the formation of the membrane attack complex, stage 3. The membrane attack complex causes lysis of bacterial organisms. In the meanwhile, C4a, C3a, and C5a peptides released during stages 1 and 2 begin the inflammatory process. See text for further details. (Adapted from Roitt et al., 1985c.)

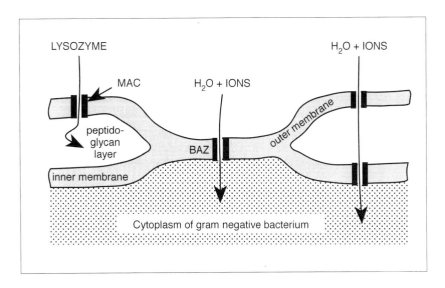

**FIGURE 8-10   The possible action of the membrane attack complex (MAC) on bacterial cell membranes.** In gram-negative organisms lysis of the outer membrane by MAC (*left*) allows lysozyme to enter and initiate hydrolysis of the peptidoglycan layer. Afterward, MAC formation takes place at the inner membrane (*right*). This allows water and ions to enter the bacterium and cause its lysis. Alternately, MACs may form at limited regions where the outer and inner membranes are fused, the Bayer adhesion zones (BAZ). Since there are no intervening peptidoglycans, membrane perforation here directly brings about bacterial lysis. The exact mechanism is unknown. (Adapted from Morgan, 1991.)

This complex forms a channel in the antigen membrane through which sodium ions and water molecules quickly pass. The formation of the channel and rapid movement of water and ions cause lysis of gram-negative bacterial membranes due to the osmotic shock produced by the lesion. An additional mechanism is that the channel allows the entrance of lysozyme, which attacks the thinner peptidoglycan wall between the outer lipoprotein cover and the plasma membrane of the bacteria (Morgan, 1991) as shown in Figure 8-10. *Viruses exposed to complement are neutralized, but osmotic stress is not a factor.* That is, complement prevents a virus from attaching to host cells by covering the viral surface with complement proteins. The fate of the C5a fragment, mentioned before, is similar to that of the C3a fragment, and this is discussed below.

## Inflammation

Inflammation is a physiological reaction to an injury or an invasion by foreign antigens, but it uses biochemical mechanisms. The process of inflammation consists of a series of biochemical reactions that include three physiological events: (1) increased blood supply to the affected area; (2) increased capillary permeability, which allows white blood cells (leucocytes) and many large molecules to enter the interstitial spaces; and (3) migration of leucocytes to the exact site of the injury of foreign invasion (chemotaxis). The migration is accompanied by phagocytosis of foreign matter by the leucocytes. Complement fixation provides the biochemical agents for this process to occur, but other biochemical substances can also control this process. Three complement peptides, which are formed during complement fixation (or activation), are involved: C4a, C3a, and C5a. These peptides, which are formed by the protein hydrolytic reactions mentioned previously, are also referred to as *anaphylatoxins* because their injection (in pure form) into animals can produce a lethal immune reaction similar to the anaphylactic shock that can occur in hypersensitive individuals (Bach, 1982). Of the three, C5a is the most powerful, since it is resistant to inactivation by serum carboxypeptidase N, an enzyme that removes a critical C-terminal Arg from each peptide. These peptides diffuse away from the site of complement fixation until they encounter local blood vessels and mast cells. Mast cells are small white blood cells that, like basophils, contain numerous granules. The granules hold inflammatory agents, including histamine, serotonin, prostaglandins, leucotrienes (substances related in structure to prostaglandins, see Chapter 6), and platelet-activating factor. The complement peptides mentioned bind to the mast cell surface at receptor proteins, which inhibit the activity of adenylate cyclase (after binding). Whether a $G_I$ protein intermediate is involved is not certain. However, this mechanism is very similar to that used by local hormones (Chapter 6). Internally, the decreased activity of adenylate cyclase lowers the levels of cAMP (since the phosphodiesterase is unaffected). Lower levels of cAMP cause the mast cell granules to fuse with the plasma membrane and release their contents into the tissue environment (Figure 8-11).

At this point, the released histamine as well as other C4–3-5a peptides (not involved in binding to mast cells) diffuse toward local blood vessels, where they induce vasodilation, an increase in the diameter of blood vessels. This, in turn, increases the local blood supply, allows fluid to leak from the vessels, and causes white blood cells to adhere to the blood vessel walls (pavementing) and to squeeze through the wall itself into the surrounding interstitial fluid, diapedesis (from the Greek *diapēdan*, to jump through). The biochemical mechanism for this process is not understood. Once released, the leucocytes (white blood cells) are guided to the site of the immune reaction (complement fixation) by the chemical gradient created by the diffusing C4–3-5a peptides. This is the process of *chemotaxis*. Although this mechanism has not yet been described satisfactorily, it may be hypothesized that the direction in which the leucocytes travel is determined by the number and location of C4–3-5a peptides bound to receptor proteins on a given region of the leucocyte membrane (Figure 8-12).

Upon arrival at the site of complement fixation where the offending antigens are present, it is necessary that the leucocyte be able to recognize the antigen (or antigen particles if the membrane attack complex [MAC] has destroyed any bacteria). The coating these antigens receive from the binding of antibody (IgG) and complement protein components represents a process called: *opsonization* (Greek *opsōnein*, prepared for dinner). The process identifies the antigens as targets for the leucocytes. Leucocytes possess receptor proteins for these opsonization components and after binding to them, begin an interesting transformation. The antigens are surrounded by the leucocyte membranes and internalized. Then the membrane-enclosed antigens fuse with lysosomes and the antigenic particles (or even whole

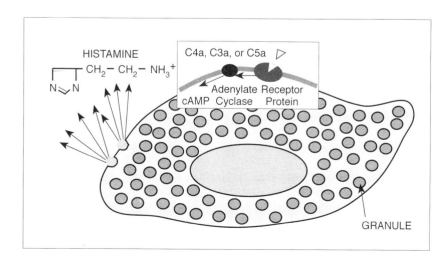

**FIGURE 8-11   Mast cell degranulation.**
C4a, C3a, or C5a peptides bind to receptor proteins on the cell's plasma membrane. This action inhibits adenylate cyclase activity and lowers the levels of cAMP. Lower levels of cAMP cause granules to fuse with the cell membrane and release their contents of histamine and other inflammatory reactants.

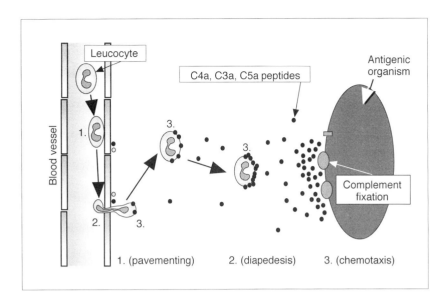

**FIGURE 8-12    Leucocyte migration toward an antigen during the inflammatory response.**
Histamine and complement inflammatory peptides cause white blood cells (*leucocyte*) to adhere to blood vessel walls (pavementing) and then to be transported through the wall (diapedesis) and migrate to the antigen (chemotaxis).

bacteria or viruses) and are destroyed. Several mechanisms are employed in this process. In the fused phagosome and lysosome organelle (phagolysosome), approximately 40 hydrolytic enzymes act to break down the viral or bacterial structures (Alberts et al., 1989a). These enzymes include proteases, nucleases, glycosidases, lipases, phospholipases, phosphatases, and sulfatases. All these enzymes function maximally at approximately pH 5.0, and the interior of the phagolysosome is maintained near that pH by a proton pump ($H^+$-ATPase) at the organelle membrane. In another mechanism, it has been suggested that the pH environment inside the phagolysosome is temporarily made alkaline so that certain cationic proteins may further damage the outer lipid layer of gram-negative bacteria (Roitt et al., 1985a; Griffin, 1988). Afterward, the pH drops to 5, so that the hydrolytic enzymes may attack the bacterial contents (Figure 8-13). The coup de grace, however, is administered by the leucocyte's use of destructive forms of oxygen through a process known as the *respiratory burst*.

The respiratory burst is actually "turned on" prior to the engulfment of the offending antigenic substance (bacterium, virus, or other invader). Boggiolini and Wymann (1990) have explained that the initial product, the

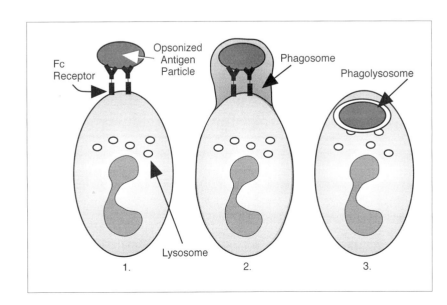

**FIGURE 8-13    Phagocytosis of opsonized antigens by leucocytes.**
The Fc receptor protein is one that will bind to the stem of an antibody. In stage 1 the leucocyte binds to the antigen. In stage 2 it forms a compartmentalized organelle around the antigen (phagosome) and moves the phagosome inward. In stage 3 lysosomes fuse with the phagosome, contributing their lytic enzymes to form a phagolysosome.

superoxide anion, is made by NADPH oxidase almost immediately as the antigenic substance is bound to the surface of the leucocyte. This destructive anion is released at either the outer surface of the plasma membrane of the leucocyte or in the newly formed phagosome itself. Eventually, even more powerful forms of oxygen radicals, such as ·OH (hydroxide radical) and the ·OCl (hypochlorite radical) are formed, which attack and destroy membrane lipids and proteins indiscriminately (Griffin, 1988) (Figure 8-14). This process may become so strong as to cause the eventual destruction of the leucocytes themselves and some of the immediately surrounding healthy cells. It also is largely responsible for the formation of tissue debris (pus) in an inflammatory reaction.

## Ocular Complement and Inflammation

Complement fixation is normally restricted to the ocular surface since the Clq protein (410 kd) is too large to penetrate the cornea and none of the complement proteins are transported into the aqueous chamber and the interstitial fluids of the retina. *Staphylococcus aureus*, one of the most common ocular pathogens, is a gram-positive organism whose destruction is actually enhanced by complement fixation prior to phagocytosis (Friedlander, 1993). It is important to emphasize here that even though the MAC components of complement are unable to destroy the organism, they are opsonized by complement before they are destroyed. Other bacterial organisms that may elicit complement reactions on the ocular surface include *Neisseria gonorrhoeae* and *Haemophilus influenzae* (two gram-negative organisms). In viral infections, herpes simplex seems to cause a complement reaction only when the virus penetrates to the stromal level. That is, it occurs when the number of antibodies is great enough to cause complement fixation to occur. In some diseases, complement fixation followed by phagocytosis fails completely. An ocular example is histoplasmosis, a disease caused by *Histoplasma capsulatum*, a yeastlike fungus. Fungi are plant organisms. In eyes involved with histoplasmosis, anterior segment inflammation is absent and neutrophils are unable to kill the fungi, though it is known that the organisms become covered with antibodies. Friedlander (1993) has indicated that the neutrophils do not become activated. It may be that the

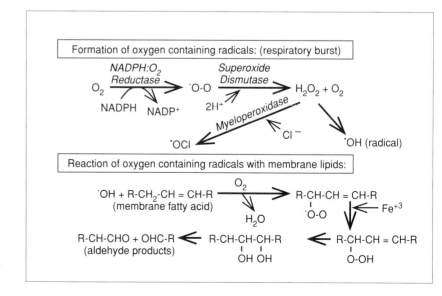

**FIGURE 8-14** Formation of three free radicals by respiratory burst: superoxide (·O—O), hydroxyl radical (·OH), and hypochlorite radical (·OCl).

These radicals combine (for example) with membrane fatty acids in combination with oxygen and ferric ion to produce aldehyde products that destroy membranes.

organism secretes molecules that either block inflammation and chemo-taxis or prevent phagocytosis. Such antiimmune mechanisms are known to occur in certain species of bacteria (Roitt et al., 1985a).

## Summary

Molecular mechanisms of immunity are principally involved in antigen-antibody reactions, complement formation, and the inflammatory re-sponse. Although there are other molecular interactions, they are generally considered to be cell-mediated events. There are five major classes of im-munoglobulins: IgA, IgD, IgE, IgG, and IgM. Generally, only classes A, G, and M are involved in ocular defense. Of these, IgA functions predomi-nately in the secretory forms and IgM is limited to the ocular surface, due to its large size. The immunoglobulins are made by B lymphocytes and are specifically designed to interact with an antigenic region of one or very few invading foreign substances or organisms. The immunoglobulins coat an antigen's surface and prepare it for complement activation and, possibly, phagocytosis. They may also prevent the antigen from attaching to or in-vading host cells. In the eye, immunoglobulins are not found in the deeper regions (i.e., lens, vitreous, retina). Complement is a series of proteins that interact to coat bacterial, viral, and fungal surfaces, in order to either destroy them or prepare them (opsonization) for engulfment by white blood cells (phagocytosis). Complement fixation releases peptides in the interstitial fluid (or precorneal tear film), to attract white blood cells to the site of antigen invasion (chemotaxis). Some bacteria are known to activate com-plement fixation in the eye.

## References

Alberts B, Bray D, Lewis J, Raff M, Roberts K, and Watson JD. *Molecular Biology of the Cell*, 2nd ed. New York, Garland, 1989a;459–461.

Alberts B, Bray D, Lewis J, Raff M, Roberts K, and Watson JD. *Molecular Biology of the Cell*, 2nd ed. New York, Garland, 1989b;1022.

Allansmith MR, Whitney CR, McLellan BH, and Newman LP. Immunoglo-bulins in the human eye. *Arch Ophthalmol* 1973;89:36–45.

Bach J-F. *Immunology*, 2nd ed. New York, John Wiley & Sons, 1982;266:127–155.

Banchereau J, and Rousset F. Human B lymphocytes: Phenotype, prolifer-ation, and differentiation. *Adv Immunol* 1992;52:125–262.

Berson SA, and Yalow RS. General principles of radioimmunoassay. *Clin Chim Acta* 1968;22:51–69.

Boggiolini M, and Wymann MP. Turning on the respiratory burst. *Trends Biochem Sci* 1990;15:69–72.

Day ED. *Advanced Immunochemistry*, 2nd ed. New York, Wiley-Liss, 1990;4–6.

Friedlander M. *Allergy and Immunology of the Eye.* New York, Raven, 1993;109–133.

Fullard RJ, and Tucker DL. Changes in human tear protein levels with progressively increasing stimulus. *Invest Ophthalmol Vis Sci* 1991;32:2290–2301.

Griffin FM. Opsonization, phagocytosis and intracellular microbial killing. *In* Rother K, and Till GO (eds). *The Complement System.* Berlin, Springer-Verlag, 1988;397–418.

Lam SKA, and Reid KBM. *Complement.* Oxford, IRL, 1988;21–22.

McBride BW, and Ward KA. Herpes simplex–specific IgG subclass response in herpetic keratitis. *J Med Virol* 1987; 21:179–189.

Morgan BP. *Complement, Clinical Aspects and Relevance to Disease.* London, Academic, 1991;38–39:104–107.

Nisonoff A. *Introduction to Molecular Immunology,* 2nd ed. Sunderland, Mass: Sinauer 1985;20–22.

Roitt I, Brostoff J, and Male D. *Immunology.* St. Louis: CV Mosby, 1985a; 5.7, 16.8–16.10.

Roitt I, Brostoff J, and Male D. *Immunology.* St. Louis: CV Mosby, 1985b; 5.1–5.5.

Roitt I, Brostoff J, and Male D. *Immunology.* St. Louis: CV Mosby, 1985c; 7.1–7.9.

Silverman LM, Christenson RH, and Grant GH. Amino acids and proteins. *In* Tietz NW (ed). *Textbook of Clinical Chemistry,* Philadelphia: WB Saunders, 1986;566–573.

Smolin G, and O'Connor GR. *Ocular Immunology*, 2nd ed. Boston, Little, Brown, 1986;7–12.

Wall JR, Salvi M, and Bernard N. Eye disease and autoimmune thyroid disorders: mechanisms for the association. *In* Wall JR and How J (eds). *Graves' Opthalmology.* Boston, Blackwell Scientific, 1990; 63–77.

Zachau HG. Immunoglobulin light-chain genes of the κ type in man and mouse. *In* Jonjio T, Alt FW, and Rabbits TH (eds). *Immunoglobulin Genes.* New York, Academic Press, 1989;91–109.

# GLOSSARY

**Action potential**   A moving wave of depolarization through a nerve caused by rapid lateral transport of sodium and potassium ions through its membranes.

**Active site**   Location on an enzyme where a catalytic reaction takes place.

**Aggregate**   A collection of proteins whose conformation and bonding are not well defined.

**Allosteric enzyme**   An enzyme whose activity is influenced by substances that bind at alternate sites (see Chapter 2).

**Amino acid**   An acid containing at least one amino group ($NH_2$) linked to the carbon atom (COOH; $\alpha$ carbon) adjacent to its carboxylic acid.

**Amphipathic**   Compound that has literally, *two characteristics*. A compound that has a hydrophobic (not compatible with water) region and a hydrophilic (compatible with water) region.

**Antibody**   A protein, also known as an immunoglobulin, that usually reacts with a foreign molecule (antigen) within body tissues and fluids (see Chapter 8).

**ATP (adenosine triphosphate) synthase**   The enzyme in the mitochondrion that converts adenosine diphosphate (ADP) to ATP and releases it when a proton passes through its structure.

**Autonomic nervous system (ANS)**   The part of the nervous system that is under involuntary control (control coming from either the brain or the spinal cord). The ANS controls a variety of physiological functions in the eye, including pupil size, accommodation, intraocular pressure, and regulation of blood flow. The sympathetic and parasympathetic divisions of the ANS tend to control opposing functions (e.g., one dilates the pupil and the other constricts it), but there are many exceptions.

**Bleaching of rhodopsin**   Conversion of rhodopsin to opsin plus all-*trans* retinal.

**Carbohydrate**   A polyhydroxy compound with the general formula $C_n(H_2O)_n$ that may have other functional groups, such as a carbonyl group. *Sugar* and *saccharide* are alternate terms.

**Cataract**   Any opacity in the lens that alters vision.

**Ceramide**   The compound formed when a fatty acid is esterified to sphingosine (see Figure 4-12).

**Chaperone**   A protein that tends to renature denatured proteins (i.e., return them to their normal conformation).

**Chromosome**   A single molecule of DNA. At metaphase a "chromosome" is actually two chromosomes (chromatids) bound together.

**Coenzyme**   Another name for a second substrate.

**Collagen**   An extracellular protein that gives structural support to tissues. Thirteen different types exist.

**Collagen fiber**   A structural edifice of collagen that is made up of several fibrils (10 to 300 nm diameter). Fibrils are composed of microfibrils, each of which is composed of five rows of tropocollagen units of undefined length.

**Comparative metabolism**   The process in which different forms of metabolism are contrasted and measured to note their advantage to each cell type.

**Condensation reaction**   The formation of a larger compound from two smaller compounds (also known as *ligation*).

**Cone transducing proteins**   Proteins similar to rhodopsin that are found in cone photoreceptors.

**Crystallins**   Proteins characteristic of the crystalline lens. There are three major classes in the adult human eye.

**Dark current**   The flow of sodium ions into and out of photoreceptors, which is maximal in the dark.

**Denaturation**   In reference to proteins, this is the process in which proteins lose their function by an alteration in their structure.

**Deoxyribonucleic acid (DNA)**   A genetic molecule which preserves the genome of a cell. It consists of four kinds of bases, as well as deoxyribose and phosphate. The phosphate imparts acidity to the molecule.

**Diabetes**   A disease that results in the unequal distribution of glucose inside and outside of cells as a result of the inability of certain cells to transport glucose efficiently.

**Diester**   Literally, any compound having two ester bonds. In the precorneal tear film it refers to any bonding combination of three precursor molecules: hydroxy fatty acid, long-chain alcohol, and cholesterol.

**Disulfide bond**   The chemical bond that connects two sulfur atoms and acts as a bridge between the same or different polypeptides. The bond occurs between two cysteine amino acids.

**DNA mutation**   Any alteration in DNA (such as the formation of a pyrimidine dimer) that causes an aberrant function of DNA.

**Domain**   A functional region of a polypeptide.

**Endocrine cells**   Cells that secrete chemical substances into the bloodstream.

**Enzyme**   A protein catalyst. (The term means *in yeast*, where enzymes were first discovered.)

**Enzyme-substrate complex (ES)**   An enzyme having a substrate at its active site.

**Extension peptides**   Nonhelical portions of collagen that are lysed or broken off in some collagen types with the formation of tropocollagen.

**Fat**   A lipid ester of fatty acid and glycerol.

**Fat-soluble vitamin**   A lipid that acts as a vitamin.

**Feedback inhibition**   Inhibition of an enzyme by a product formed along a metabolic pathway in which the enzyme participates.

**G proteins**   Proteins that normally bind guanosine diphosphate (GDP) when inactive but that when stimulated by a receptor protein bind guanosine triphosphate (GTP). They are intermediates between receptor proteins and enzymes that synthesize or degrade second messengers. G proteins either activate or inhibit these enzymes.

**Galactosemia**   A disease involving the inability of cells to metabolize galactose as a result of a deficiency of one of three enzymes.

**Ganglioside**   A compound formed when more than one carbohydrate is bound to ceramide (see Figure 4-13).

**Gate protein**   A type of transport protein that allows only specific substances (usually ions) to cross a plasma membrane by facilitated diffusion. During action potentials two different gate proteins for sodium and potassium ions are operative. These proteins are also called channel proteins or voltage-dependent gate proteins. In the postsynaptic membrane, a sodium ion channel receptor protein (nicotinic receptor) belongs to a group of channel proteins that are ligand- or neurotransmitter activated.

**Gel**   A homogeneously dispersed solid within a liquid, which is viscous in nature.

**Genetic code**   A series of three base sequences in nucleic acids that code for amino acids as well as for the initiation and halting of protein synthesis.

**Genome**   The entire genetic information contained within a cell.

**Glycolysis**   Literally, *splitting of carbohydrates*. The term is synonymous with the Embden-Meyerhof pathway, a process that ends with the formation of pyruvate. Glycolysis can be either anaerobic or aerobic, depending upon the metabolic fate of pyruvate.

**Glycosaminoglycans (GAGs)**   Carbohydrate polymers composed of disaccharide units of one amino sugar and one nonamino sugar. They have a high density of negative charges.

**Haworth structure**   A convention used to represent carbohydrates in a ring structure (named after Sir W. N. Haworth, who won the Nobel prize for his contribution in establishing that glucose exists in solution predominately in a ring form); see Figures 3-2, 3-3.

**Histone**   A basic protein that binds to DNA in order to compact it within the cellular nucleus.

**Hormone**   A chemical messenger, belonging to several classes, that is released either from cell to cell in the bloodstream (or the interstitial fluid) or within a single cell. Originally, a hormone was only considered to be a substance that was released from a cell and delivered via the bloodstream to another cell. That restricted concept is now outdated.

**Hormone response**   The physiological response to a hormone that is brought about either by a biochemical receptor–second messenger cascade or by a biochemical receptor–enhancer interaction. The first mechanism activates several enzymes in sequence, whereas the second either promotes or inhibits protein synthesis at the DNA level.

**Horner's syndrome**   A lesion in a sympathetic autonomic nerve that results in reduced pupil size and causes the eyelid to droop on the affected side.

**Hydrogen bond**   A relatively weak bond between a hydrogen atom and an atom of oxygen or nitrogen. Such bonds are temporary, but their number can be quite large and influential in the stability of a compound. They occur very often between water and their solutes, within protein structures, and in nucleic acids.

**Hydrolysis reaction**   Cleavage of a compound by the addition of a water molecule.

**Hydrophobic**   The property of being lipid soluble or soluble in organic solvents. The name literally means *water huting* or *water fearing*.

**Hyperpolarization**   Increase in the negative charge within a cell.

**Indoleamine**   Another name for serotonin, a neurotransmitter. It is derived from the amino acid tryptophan.

**Inhibition**   The process of decreasing the normal velocity of an enzyme-catalyzed reaction with an inhibitor substance.

**Integral protein**   A protein that enters or crosses a bilipid membrane, also known as an *intrinsic membrane protein*.

**Isomerization**   Relocation of a portion of a molecule to a different site on the same molecule.

**Isozyme**   One of several different polypeptide sequences of the same enzyme that have kinetic properties. *Isoform* is an alternate term.

**$K_{apparent}$**   ($K_{app}$ or $K_{0.5}$) The concentration of substrate at which $V_{max}$ is one-half its normal value. It is used for enzymes that do not follow Michaelis-Menten kinetics and have no absolute $K_m$ value and for Michaelis-Menten enzymes in the presence of an inhibitor.

**$K_I$**   Inhibitor constant that is equivalent to the $K_m$ for a substrate. It is an indirect measure of the affinity of an inhibitor for an enzyme.

**$K_m$**   Michaelis-Menten constant that is equivalent to $k_2/k_1$ (with $k_3$ sufficiently small) or to the concentration of a substrate at which $V_m$ is one-half its normal value.

**Ketone bodies**   Acidic metabolites of fatty acids formed from their excessive catabolism (that occur, e.g., in more severe forms of diabetes).

**Lipid**   A class of nonprotein compounds that are predominately hydrophobic but which have hydrophilic moieties or parts.

**Lipophilic**   Lipid-soluble, literally *fat-loving*.

**Masking**   The biochemical alteration of the N-terminal end of a protein to prevent its degradation. In cells this is often accomplished by adding acetyl groups.

**Metabolism**   The sum total of the chemical reactions that occur in cells. Anabolic reactions are involved with synthesis while catabolic reactions are concerned with degradation and the generation of energy.

**Metal chelation**   Binding of metals (such as iron, copper, cobalt) by surrounding the metal with a cagelike structure.

**Michaelis-Menten enzyme**   An enzyme whose activity is governed by Michaelis-Menten kinetics (see Chapter 2).

**Mitochondrion**   (plural: mitochondria) A subcellular organelle in which certain metabolic processes (especially oxidative phosphorylation described in Chapter 3) are isolated from the remainder of the cell.

**Motif**   A subset of a domain. Two or more motifs may form a domain, but not a complete polypeptide.

**Mucins**   Mucus glycoproteins found principally in the mucoid layer of the precorneal tear film.

**Nucleoside**   A nitrogenous ring compound (base) bound to a pentose.

**Nucleotide**   A base bound to a pentose plus one or more phosphates.

**Oxidation-reduction reaction**   A chemical reaction in which electrons are transferred from one substance (oxidation reaction) to another (reduction reaction).

**Paracrine cells**   Cells that secrete chemical substances only to the immediately surrounding tissue including the cells that release the substance.

**Partial pressure**   Usually indicated by a small "p" in front of a gas, it represents the pressure exerted by a gas (in a mixture of gases) as if it were present alone in a container or a given tissue.

**Peptidoglycan**   A polymer composed of peptides and sugar derivatives.

**Peripheral protein**   A protein that is attached to a bilipid membrane but does not enter it.

**Phosphorylation**   The process of adding a phosphate group to a compound or metabolic intermediate. In the generation of high-energy adenosine triphosphate (ATP) phosphorylation can be either simple (substrate level) or complex (oxidative). In the latter case, electron and proton transports are involved (see Chapter 3).

**pI**   (isoelectric point). The pH at which all of the positive and negative charges on a protein or other molecule are equal.

**Polymerase**   (an enzyme that synthesizes nucleic acids). There are several types: a DNA-directed DNA polymerase makes DNA from a DNA template. DNA-directed RNA polymerases make RNA from a DNA template. Viruses use other types as well.

**Polyols**   Polyhydroxy intermediates formed in the polyol pathway, which are a source of osmotic stress for cells, especially those of the lens.

**Postsynaptic inhibition**   The process in which nerve conduction in the postsynaptic nerve or muscle cell is presented. This may be increased hyperpolarization of that cell. The term *inhibitory postsynaptic potential* (IPSP) is also used. An IPSP may be caused by an inhibitory neurotransmitter or by a decrease in the amount of neurotransmitters released across the cleft (as occurs with cone photoreceptors).

**Postsynaptic stimulation**   The process in which nervous transmission or depolarization is continued in the postsynaptic nerve or muscle cell. The term *excitatory postsynaptic potential* (EPSP) is also used. However, note that in photoreceptor cells (and in some bipolar cells) an EPSP is caused by presynaptic hyperpolarization that stops the release of neurotransmitters.

**Posttranslational modification**   The biochemical alteration of a protein after the synthesis of its polypeptide chain.

**Protein**   Polymer of amino acids linked by peptide bonds, usually with a molecular weight of 10 kd or more.

**Protein structure**   There are several divisions: *Primary:* amino acid sequence; *secondary:* unique shapes of part of the sequence (α-helices, β-pleated sheets, turns, random coils); *tertiary:* conformation of a single polypeptide; *quaternary:* conformation of two or more polypeptides that comprise one protein. A domain is an intermediary form between secondary and tertiary structure.

**Proteoglycan**   The complex that results from the binding of a glycosaminoglycan (GAG) to a protein.

**Pyrimidine dimers**   Two adjacent pyrimidine bases on the same DNA chain that have a common bond.

**Quantitative Schirmer 1 test**   This is a quantitative test that was described by Van Bijsterveld in 1974. Most Schirmer tests are qualitative when used clinically.

**Rate-limiting enzyme**   An enzyme that governs the formation of products in one direction. Its rate of catalysis is usually slower than that of other enzymes in a pathway.

**Replication**   The process of making new DNA from old DNA.

**Retinal**   Vitamin A aldehyde, the prosthetic group bound in opsin to form rhodopsin.

**Retinitis pigmentosa**   A degeneration of the retinal neural cells. Its cause is unknown.

**Rhodopsin**   Rod pigment protein that contains 11-*cis* retinal and is involved in the initial phase of phototransduction.

**Ribonucleic acid (RNA)**   A genetic molecule that is involved in supplying the code for protein synthesis. It is similar to DNA but substitutes uracil for thymine and ribose for deoxyribose. (See Chapter 5 for types.)

**S (Svedberg unit)**   This is a sedimentation coefficient used in high-speed or ultracentrifugation. It is roughly proportional to particle mass and is used when the molecular weight is unknown. S is the specific volume, in milliliters per gram, of the particle divided by the product of the angular velocity per second and the rate in revolutions per minute.

**Saccharide**   See *carbohydrate.*

**Saturation**   This term refers to the amount of double bonds present in a compound. The presence of a single double-bond makes the compound unsaturated. A completely saturated compound has no double bonds.

**Schiff base**   ($R_1$—CH = $NH^+$—$R_2$) It is a bond which exists between retinal and opsin. The bond is protonated in rhodopsin and is somewhat weak for a covalent bond.

**Second messenger**   An internal cell hormone: cyclic adenosine monophosphate (cAMP), cyclic guanosine monophosphate (cGMP), calcium ion, or a phosphoinositide.

**Sphingomyelin**   The compound formed when a phosphocholine is esterified to ceramide (see Chapter 4 and Figure 4-12).

**Sphingosine**   A long-chain dihydroxy amino alcohol used to form glycolipids (see Chapter 4 and Figure 4-11).

**Substrate**   A substance or metabolite that is converted to a product by an enzyme.

**Sulfoxide bond**   A bond formed between sulfur and oxygen in the amino acid methionine found in proteins (see Chapter 1 and Figure 1-13). It accompanies disulfide bond formation in crystallins.

**Target tissues (target cells)**   Tissues whose cells have receptor proteins either at their plasma membranes or in their cytoplasm for specific endocrine or paracrine hormones.

**Transcription**   The process of making RNA from DNA. *Reversed transcription* is the formation of DNA from RNA as occurs in some viruses.

**Transducin**   The G protein of photoreceptors that is stimulated by rhodopsin.

**Translation**   The process of protein synthesis from mRNA.

**Tropocollagen**   The essential triple helical unit of collagen. It is formed extracellularly; see Chapter 1.

**Unsaturation**   See *saturation.*

**Upstream promoter**   A region of DNA on the 3' side of one or more genes that controls transcription of that gene by DNA-directed RNA polymerase.

**v (Velocity)**   The *velocity of a reaction* is the reaction rate of enzyme catalyzed reactions, and is usually expressed as moles of substrate used or product formed per unit time. For Michaelis-Menten kinetics, the velocity equation (2–4, in Chapter 2) is derived as follows:

Since: $k_1 [E][S] - (k_2[ES] + k_3[ES]) = 0$,
   when $d[ES]/dt = 0$
   $k_1[E][S] = (k_2 + k_3) [ES]$
   then $\dfrac{[E][S]}{[ES]} = \dfrac{k_2 + k_3}{k_1}$
   where $k_2 + k_3/k_1 = K_m$ (Michaelis-Menten constant)
   And $[E] = [E_0] - [ES]$
   where $[E_0] =$ Enzyme concentration at $t = 0$.
   and $\dfrac{([E_0] - [ES])\,[S]}{[ES]} = K_m$
   by rearrangement: $\dfrac{[E_0][S]}{K_m + [S]} = [ES]$.
Since the velocity of a reaction is also
   $v = k_3[ES]$
By substitution, $v = \dfrac{k_3[E_0][S]}{K_m + [S]}$
The maximal velocity of the reaction:
   $V_{max} = k_3[E_0]$
Therefore, the Michaelis-Menten velocity of a reaction is
   $v = \dfrac{V_{max}[S]}{K_m + [S]}$

**V$_{max}$**   This is the maximum velocity of an enzyme-catalyzed reaction that is possible.

**Virus**   An organism composed of a nucleic acid (DNA or RNA) and a capsid (protein coat) that must enter a cell to reproduce itself. In the process, it eventually kills the host cell by manipulating the genetic machinery of the cell for its own purpose.

**Vitamin**   A substance that is essential for biological metabolism in higher organisms but one that the organisms cannot make. There are two classes, lipid-soluble and water-soluble vitamins.

**Vitrosin**   Collagen found in the vitreous. It is type II collagen to which is attached type IX.

**Wax**   An ester made up of a fatty acid and a long-chain alcohol.

**X-ray crystallography**   The determination of the three-dimensional structure of compounds using x-rays to produce a diffraction pattern from a crystal of a pure compound.

# Index

Page numbers followed by *t* and *f* indicate tables and figures, respectively. Page numbers in **boldface** indicate terms defined in the Glossary.

Hydrolysis, 39–42
Hydrolysis reaction, **185**
Hydrophilic compound, definition of, 87
Hydrophobic compound, definition of, 87, **186**
Hyperpolarization, 154, **186**
Hyperthyroidism, 141–142
Hypervariable regions, of immunoglobulin, 168f
Hypothalamus, endocrine functions of, 131–133, 132f

IDDM. *See* Diabetes mellitus, insulin-dependent (type I)
Iduronic acid, 81, 81f
Immunochemistry, 167–181
Immunoglobulin(s), 167–173
    antigen binding
        kinetics, 171
        specificity, 172–173, 173f
    antigen-binding region, 171, 172t
    classes of, 169, 169t
    ocular, 169t, 174
    structure of, 2–3, 167
        primary, 3
        quaternary, 4
        secondary, 3
        tertiary, 4
    synthesis of, 172
Immunoglobulin A
    characteristics of, 169, 169t, 170f
    concentrations in ocular tissues, 169t, 174
    J chain, 169
    S chain, 169
    secretory, 169, 170f, 174
Immunoglobulin D
    characteristics of, 169, 169t, 170f
    concentrations in ocular tissues, 169, 169t
Immunoglobulin E
    characteristics of, 169, 169t, 170f
    concentrations in ocular tissues, 169, 169t
Immunoglobulin G
    characteristics of, 169t, 169–170, 170f
    concentrations in ocular tissues, 169, 169t, 170, 174
    response to herpes simplex invasion, 174, 175t
    structure of, 5f-6f, 6, 7f, 167, 168f
Immunoglobulin M
    characteristics of, 169t, 170, 170f
    concentrations in ocular tissues, 169t, 174
    J chain, 170
Immunology, 167
Indoleamine, **186**
    as neurotransmitter, 161
Inflammation
    biochemistry of, 177–181
    ocular, complement fixation in, 180–181
Inhibition, enzyme, 35–38, **186**
Inhibitory postsynaptic potentials, 153–154, 154f, **187**

Insulin, 132f, 133t
    actions of, 74
    amino acid sequence, 74f
    receptors, 75, 76f
    structure of, 74, 74f
Insulin-dependent cells
    altered metabolism in, in diabetes, 75
    types of, 75
Interplexiform cell, in retinal light reception, 162
Intraocular pressure
    generation of, 31, 44
    modulation of, 158
        eicosanoid effects on, 147
        steroid effects on, 145
Intrinsic (integral) membrane proteins, 96, 97f
Introns, 116–117, 117f
Ion channels, in neurotransmission, 151–153, 152f-153f
Ion transport, in neurotransmission, 151, 152f, 152–153, 153f
Iris, blood flow through, 73t
Isomerization, **186**
Isoprene, in isoprenoids, 91–92, 92f
Isoprenoids, 91–92
Isozyme, definition of, 46

J gene, 173, 173f

$K_{apparent}$ ($K_{app}$ or $K_{0.5}$), 35, 36f, **186**
Keratan sulfate, 81f, 81–82
Keratin, in meibomian gland dysfunction, 99
Keratoconjunctivitis sicca, quantitative Schirmer 1 test in, 42
Keratomalacia, 102
Ketone bodies, **186**
    production, 75, 75f
$K_I$, 35–38, **186**
$K_m$, 33–34, 34f, **186**
Krebs cycle, 58, 59f, 63–64, 64f
Kühne, Willy, 16

Lactate dehydrogenase, 44–48, 155
    in cornea, isozyme density patterns, 47, 47f
    isozymes, 45–47
    in lens, isozyme density patterns, 47f, 47–48
    reaction catalyzed by, 45, 45f
    in retina, 48
    structure of, 45–46, 46f
Lactose, structure of, 54–55, 56f
Laminin, molecular weight, 7t
Lens
    carbohydrate metabolism in, 71t, 71–73
    development of, 122f, 122–123
    in diabetes, 77
    epithelial cells, carbohydrate metabolism in, 71t, 72

fiber cells, production, 72
focus, regulation of, 156
LDH isozyme density patterns in, 47f, 47–48
proteins
    in cataract formation, 12, 12f
    structural, 9
    yellowing, with aging, 15
Lens capsule, collagen in, 26
Leucocytes (white blood cells)
    chemotaxis, 177–178, 179f
    diapedesis, 178, 179f
    in inflammation, 177–178, 179f
    pavementing, 178, 179f
    respiratory burst, 179–180, 180f
Leucotriene(s), 146
    paracrine effects of, 146
Leucotriene $E_4$, 137t
Lid retraction, in hyperthyroidism, 141–142, 144
Ligation, 32
Light transduction, 139f, 139–141, 141f, 159–162
Lineweaver-Burk plot
    of allosteric enzyme, 35, 37f
    of Michaelis-Menten enzyme, 34, 35f
        with inhibition, 35, 37f, 38, 38f
Lipids, 58, 87–104. *See also* Eicosanoids; Esters; Fatty acids; Glycolipids; Isoprenoids; Phospholipids; Triacylglycerols; Vitamin A
    amphipathic, 87
    in cell membranes, 95–97, 97f, 98t
    classification of, 87
    definition of, **186**
    versus fats, 87
    hydrophilicity, 87
    hydrophobicity, 87
    meibomian gland, composition of, 98t
    polar, 87
    precorneal tear film, 97–99, 99f
    retinal, 99–100
Lipoamide, 46t, 63
Lipophilic, definition of, **186**
Lipoxygenase, 146
Lumican, 82, 83f
Luteinizing hormone, 132f
Lysosomes, 118
Lysozyme, 38–42
    active site, 39–40, 40f
    activity, 39–40, 40f
    bactericidal activity, 38–42, 177, 177f
    catalytic mechanism, 39–42, 41f
    as indicator of tear dysfunction, 42, 42f
    molecular weight, 7t
    properties of, 39–40, 40f
    in tear film, 39

Macular edema, 147
Malate-aspartate shuttle, 66–67
Maltose, structure of, 54, 56f